Heal Thyself: Embracing Our Natural Diet for Optimal Health

Maria Manazza

ABOUT THE BOOK

This book is dedicated to everyone that continues to challenges societal norms / traditions to undertake their own healing journey despite standing out from the crowd. We are all inspired by your unwavering efforts, perseverance and determination to be your own doctor. May this book be a guiding light and empower you in the pursuit of a healthy and happy life.

To my awake family members, you hold a special place in my heart. I will always be grateful for your presence in my life, you know who you are, and I love each and every one of you.

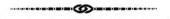

Table of Contents

ABOUT THE AUTHOR

Maria Manazza, a dedicated advocate for sustainable living and a passionate steward of the land, is a devoted practitioner of planting food forests, seed collecting, growing plants, and gardening. Born on June 7, 1978, in Langley, B.C., Canada, Maria developed her deep connection with nature and plants while growing up in Cloverdale, BC, under the loving guidance of her father, who single-handedly raised three girls.

Her journey towards a life dedicated to nurturing the earth and fostering a harmonious relationship with nature began when her family relocated to the picturesque Sunshine Coast, specifically Gibson's BC, in 1990. There, she completed her high school education at Elphinstone Secondary School, gaining a profound appreciation for the natural beauty of the region.

Maria continued her education by pursuing her passion for horticulture, studying it from 2005 to 2006 at Capilano College located in North Vancouver BC. This marked the formal beginning of her journey into the world of plants and agriculture.

In 2017, she furthered her expertise by obtaining a Detoxification Specialist Certificate from The International School of Detoxification, equipping her with valuable knowledge about the importance of a high fruit diet and the diet/disease connection.

Her commitment to holistic health and wellness led her to become a Health Coach, even though she holds no formal credentials in the field. Since 2016, she has been dedicated to guiding individuals towards a healthier, more balanced lifestyle.

Maria also delved into the intricate world of iridology, a field she is entirely self-taught in. Her passion for understanding the body's natural rhythms and signs has enabled her to help countless individuals on their journey to improved health.

In 2009, Maria embarked on a life-changing adventure when she and her husband moved to a 7-acre organic farm, driven by a desire to become more self-sufficient and have a direct connection to their food source. However, the challenges of farm life, the constant commitment it required, and her declining health eventually led her to transition from the farm to an orchard.

During her most challenging moments of healing and health recovery, Maria lived off the grid for a period, gaining a profound understanding of the simplicity and beauty of a life in close harmony with nature.

Today, Maria resides in the scenic Okanagan, BC, where she continues her mission of growing her own food whenever the weather permits. Her commitment to a natural and sustainable lifestyle is unwavering, and she shares her knowledge and passion through iridology readings, writing, health coaching, and health consultations.

Notably, Maria plays a significant role in the Terrain Model Diet Support Group, offering invaluable support to individuals transitioning to a natural diet for health and healing purposes.

In April 2024, Maria will celebrate a decade on her path to a healthier, more connected life. With 15 years of experience in gardening and growing food, she remains committed to planting fruit trees each year, firmly believing in the importance of caring for the land and embracing the benefits of growing one's own food. Her journey is a testament to the power of reconnecting with nature and the profound impact it can have on one's life and well-being.

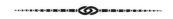

Chapter 1
Introduction

What's going on in our world? Why is there so much confusion about health and healing? Even the so-called "experts" can't agree on how to support the body's natural healing abilities or how to attain and maintain good health. There's an overwhelming amount of conflicting information and scientific studies that can be used to back up any dietary or lifestyle preference a person might have or want to try.

In a perfect world, we would instinctively know how to nourish and take care of ourselves, just like wild animals do. Our ancestors, who enjoyed vibrant health, would pass down this knowledge to us. Unfortunately, modern society has veered away from the dietary and lifestyle practices that used to keep us collectively healthy.

Nowadays, people often look for validation to support their unhealthy habits. With easy access to information, it's tempting to find content that seems to justify those choices. The internet and social media are full of wildly varying opinions on health. However, we need to keep in mind that just because information is available doesn't mean it's true. Even the experts often disagree with each other. Sadly, this confusion has led to a lack of healthy individuals among us. The overwhelming mix of contradictory advice has made it difficult for people to grasp the basics of nutrition and wellness. As a result, they feel confused and uncertain about which path to take to achieve better health.

I understand how frustrating it can be for people who just want reliable answers to their health concerns, so they can focus on what truly matters in life. Sadly, they often come across misleading or incorrect information that only adds to their confusion and keeps them unwell. Many end up relying on the medical system or on substances they believe will help them.

When we examine today's health "experts," we realize that many lack true expertise, and their recommendations can do more harm than good. The key lies in understanding the truth. To do so, we need to learn about the link between diet and disease and apply this knowledge to our own lives, seeing long-term changes that prove its effectiveness.

Regardless of what we believe, hear, read, or learn, if it's not based on truth, we cannot achieve vibrant health or effectively address our health issues. Unless we ground ourselves in truth, our thoughts, beliefs, or teachings won't help us achieve optimum health or understand and address our health issues effectively. Once we discover the truth, we must commit to applying it as a long-term lifestyle, experiencing its transformative effects firsthand. This is a separate topic worth exploring in depth.

The food we eat every day has a significant impact on our overall health. The choices we make now shape who we will become in the future. The truth remains the truth, regardless of our beliefs or actions, and nobody can escape the laws of nature and their consequences.

These laws apply to everyone, regardless of social status. It's disheartening to see the promotion, advertising, and subsidies given to foods that contribute to health issues while foods that promote good health are often expensive, inaccessible, and unfairly criticized in the media. Unfounded claims regarding sugar content in fruits is a prime example.

This book aims to equip readers with the necessary tools to tackle their health issues once and for all, guiding them through the overwhelming dietary confusion that surrounds us. It's not fair that we must spend so much time and effort worrying about whether our food choices are promoting good health or leading to illness. This book provides valuable insights and accurate dietary information to help people achieve optimal health, if they are willing to give up foods that contribute to disease and create the right conditions for their bodies to heal. Our daily choices determine our health outcomes.

Disease happens when harmful waste builds up in our bodies, causing damage and making it hard for the body to remove it effectively. This waste accumulates over time because of unhealthy foods, substances, and bad lifestyle choices. There's no easy solution or quick fix to heal from this. Like other creatures, humans thrive on a specific diet that supports their overall health. While things like toxins, accidents, and genetics can affect us, the main cause of disease is our diet and lifestyle choices. Many people experience a wide range of unpleasant symptoms, including painful periods, severe menopause symptoms, hair loss, declining eyesight, weak and brittle bones, diabetes, high blood pressure, muscle discomfort, and many more. These symptoms are often normalized and accepted as inevitable signs of getting older. However, if these symptoms were truly a natural consequence of aging, every person would experience them without exception. Surprisingly, there are individuals who don't go through such painful symptoms, challenging the belief that they are unavoidable for everyone.

We shouldn't let the daily concern of what to eat and how to heal our health issues consume us. Our purpose on this planet is to build, create, and be good stewards of the Earth. My greatest hope is that this knowledge becomes widespread and gets passed down through generations. By embracing these principles, we can empower ourselves and future generations to thrive in good health and well-being.

I don't aim to be seen as an expert on health by society. My motivation is to share information that can help improve people's health. When individuals become healthier, our world naturally becomes better too. I strongly believe that each person has the potential to achieve something remarkable in their life and positively impact others. We all have unique talents and abilities. However, when we suffer, experience pain, and struggle with maintaining good health, that potential often goes to waste.

Based on my experience as a consultant, one of the biggest challenges is helping individuals understand the simplicity of rebuilding their health amidst the unnecessary complexity that surrounds it. There are two primary reasons why achieving and maintaining good health can be difficult.

Firstly, we have been conditioned to believe that external solutions are necessary to fix our health issues, and not seeking such solutions is often seen as neglectful or ignorant. This belief undermines our ability to recognize the inherent power within ourselves to heal.

Secondly, building and maintaining good health requires a

long-term commitment and daily effort, which many people are unwilling to make. We are creatures of habit, and change can be challenging. It's natural to cling to familiar habits, hoping that our symptoms will magically disappear in the future. However, true health isn't achieved through temporary diets or superficial solutions. It requires a complete shift in lifestyle.

Unfortunately, many individuals rely on medications, supplements, and quick fixes as a shortcut to wellness. When someone manages to naturally heal themselves, they are often perceived as lucky, rather than recognizing the deliberate choices and actions they took to regain their health.

To truly rebuild our health, we must let go of the foods, substances, and lifestyle choices that contributed to our health issues in the first place. It's essential to move away from the reliance on external interventions and instead focus on nurturing our bodies through sustainable and holistic practices. Only then can we experience the true potential of our bodies to heal and thrive.

There isn't a short-term "diet" or "cleanse" that can guarantee lasting health. While following the Natural Human Diet for some time can have positive effects, it's not as simple as sticking to a specific eating pattern for a set period. Rebuilding our health takes years of applying correct knowledge, making changes to our diet and lifestyle, and addressing symptoms. Most people aren't willing to make these long-term changes because it goes against societal norms. Our habits are deeply ingrained, and change can seem overwhelming. Social pressures and lack of understanding from others make it even harder. When someone tries to adopt a healthy routine, it often meets resistance because it challenges others' habits and routines. It can be tough to take the initial steps towards change, especially when we lack energy and motivation due to illness. Some people don't want to put in the effort and prefer relying on stimulants and medications until they can't anymore. It's a sad reality that reflects the current state of our world, where being unhealthy has become the norm.

I wrote this book because I have discovered some important truths about health and healing. It took me over 9 years of trial and error to gather all the necessary information, and now I want to share it with you. People often ask me what I eat in a day and when. When I'm asked this, I realize they don't understand that what I eat today is just a small part of my overall health journey. It doesn't reflect the changes I've made over the years that have shaped my current lifestyle and eating habits. We are a product of our past and present choices. Explaining this, I emphasize that transitioning to a healthy lifestyle is as important as reaching the end goal. Each person starts from a different point, and it involves trial and error. It's crucial to stay focused on the truth and our health goals, and to commit to the daily ups and downs without giving up.

My goal is to save you time, confusion, and money, so you can focus on living your life. We shouldn't have to worry about what to eat every day or how to heal our health issues. Our purpose is to build, create, and take care of the Earth. I hope that this knowledge becomes widespread and passed down through generations.

This book goes beyond my personal opinions and experiences. It includes insights from other highly qualified experts in the health field, including medical doctors. Comparing their perspectives is enlightening and helps us understand the reasons behind their different viewpoints.

For as long as I can remember, I suffered from constant pain and health issues. At 35 years old, I hit rock bottom and realized I had to find a way to heal or face a lifetime of suffering. The medical specialist offered no solution but lifelong pain medication, which wasn't a real remedy. I had been dealing with leg pain since I was 6, and the specialist said there was no hope for healing. Feeling defeated, I couldn't accept a life filled with pain and medications. My will to find another way was stronger. Suffering often leads to two paths: giving up or taking control. I chose to take matters into my own hands and become stronger.

I strongly believe that there is always a way to achieve something if we truly desire it. This belief applied not just to health but to all aspects of life. I was determined to end my pain, feeling exhausted and tired of living with it. I hit rock bottom, which pushed me to dig deeper and find solutions. In the next chapter, I'll share my healing success story and delve into the health issues I faced and how I overcame them. If this book helps just one person find answers to their own healing, I'll consider it a success. We must heal ourselves as no one else can do it for us. It's unfair that we suffer because we were never taught how to properly care for ourselves. This vital knowledge should be passed down through generations, but instead, we've been misled about diet and human health, resulting in unnecessary suffering and disease in our world.

The great news is that once we learn the right information, we can never be misled again. The truth sticks with us, especially when it benefits us. Life shouldn't revolve solely around finding ways to alleviate pain and disease. Nowadays, it feels like everyone knows someone suffering from health issues due to misinformation and wrong choices. It's easy to doubt everything and not give this lifestyle a fair chance. We often look for shortcuts or quick fixes for results. With numerous "scientific studies" supporting various fad diets, it's tempting to try something new when things get tough. However, if we delve deep enough, we'll inevitably come back to the simple truth, whether we're ready to face it or not. Healing your health issues may not be easy, as it often involves discomfort and pain. However, continuing to live an unhealthy lifestyle can also be painful and uncomfortable. It's important to recognize that experiencing these challenges is inevitable, given that most of us were not raised with a healthy diet and environment. We have two choices: we can continue with our current lifestyle and allow toxicity to build up, leading to eventual pain and suffering, or we can start the journey to true health today. While there may be uncomfortable cleansing processes along the way, taking control of your health means experiencing these symptoms on your own terms. When we correctly take charge of our health, the body can heal itself, and that is the remedy for pain. The body heals the body when we learn how to put the correct conditions in place for it to do so.

Interestingly, I have always had a sense that I would write a book someday, although I never anticipated it would be about health and healing. Just remember, if you firmly believe in your ability to heal, have a plan for achieving it, possess the right information, and never give up despite the difficulties, success in healing is only a matter of time and patience. We all desire a better world, and the good news is that it's possible when we begin by improving our individual health. If you want to build a better world, start with yourself. Healing the body is a gradual process, and patience is a crucial asset. I want you to know that I will be repeating myself on important points throughout this book, I do so with intention, in hopes that the information will be easier to remember. I sincerely hope that the information I'm about to share in these pages will be as valuable to you as it has been to me in my own learning and life. One of my proudest achievements so far has been improving my health, as without it, I wouldn't have been able to accomplish my next great achievement: writing and completing this book.

Chapter 2
My Healing Success Story

I didn't like going to the doctor, except for emergencies or surgery, and neither did my family. Luckily, I never had to see a doctor during my childhood, or else they likely would have given me medications for the pain I experienced.

When I was 6 years old, I started having intense pain in my left leg. It kept me up at night and affected my daily life, mood, and overall well-being. The pain was excruciating, and I often found myself crying alone in the middle of the night. As a child, I didn't complain much about it, but looking back, I can see why I was sometimes cranky and mean.

In the 1990's, during my high school days, we were assembled in the cafeteria with little notice to receive the Hepatitis B vaccine. I didn't know much about vaccines at that time, so I just followed everyone else and got in line for my shot. Shortly after receiving the Hepatitis B vaccine, I blacked out and I remember being taken to the back room of our school office. I couldn't move or speak. It felt like a type of paralysis. I was surrounded by people, but I couldn't see or hear them clearly. Voices were distorted and faces were blurry. I lay there unable to function for what felt like a very long time. I was out of it for approximately 90 minutes. When I finally regained movement and function, they just sent me home since school was almost over. If I had only known, then what I know now. Isn't that often the case in life? Without knowledge, we're vulnerable. My family wasn't informed, and the incident went unreported. I never brought it up again, and I'm not sure if the school officials watching over me that day called the hospital or an ambulance while I was lying there. It was like it never happened, which I'm sure benefited everyone involved, except for me.

Looking back, I realized that around the time of the vaccine incident, my eyesight started to decline. I also lost motivation and concentration. Everything seemed to change, which affected me socially and academically. Sadly, there was nothing anyone could do for me now. Without proper knowledge, I was just another damaged face in the crowd.

In my twenties, I saw several doctors for my pain since it had been going on for too long. I didn't know much about the medical system, except that doctors were always available. After seeing multiple doctors, I was prescribed Tylenol 3s, sleeping pills, and oral birth control. One doctor admitted that he had no idea why I was in pain and referred me to a nerve specialist. Even the nerve specialist couldn't help me. He ran a few tests and concluded that I had a dead nerve in my leg. He told me I would have to take pain medication for the rest of my life.

During a trip to Italy in 2008, I experienced a sudden incident where my body including my face started tingling, and I lost my ability to talk and communicate. My whole body went numb, and I ended up sitting on the floor of a store unable to communicate. It took some time for me to regain my abilities, and although it was embarrassing, I didn't go to a hospital.

By the age of 35, my health had reached a low point. I was experiencing frequent headaches, fatigue, and other symptoms. I tried numerous natural remedies and substances, but they didn't make a significant difference. In 2009, my husband and I moved to the countryside to start an organic farm. We believed that growing our own food would help improve my health since we knew exactly where it came from and how it was produced. We followed sustainable farming methods and tried to minimize outside inputs. However, my migraine headaches worsened, leading to feelings of hopelessness and depression.

An odd incident occurred while I was living on the farm. One day, I couldn't get up from the couch and I experienced excruciating pain throughout my body. We had no idea what caused this lack of mobility. It took me several sessions with a chiropractor to restore my body to normal functioning.

These incidents reminded me of what happened in Italy, as they seemed to come out of nowhere and without warning, minus the systemic tingling and numbness.

After the incident on the couch, I started questioning my diet, which I thought was healthy because it came from our own farm. Around that time, I randomly came across a book called "The PH Miracle" by Dr. Robert Young. Reading the book made me realize that meat, dairy, and eggs were acidic foods that could cause health issues over time. It was a significant revelation, especially considering our farm lifestyle. I decided to eliminate these animal products from my diet overnight. My husband decided to join me on this journey and eventually, we decided to sell the farm. We both agreed that continuing to raise animals for food no longer aligned with our newfound knowledge.

As I removed meat, dairy, and eggs from my diet, I began to experience a sense of health and clarity in my body and my mind that I had never felt before. I discovered Arnold Ehret's book on fasting, which further enhanced my well-being when I incorporated water fasting into my routine. Later on, I learned from Dr. Robert Morse about the body's detoxification process and the importance of a high fruit diet. While Dr. Morse provided helpful information, I realized that it wasn't the complete path to wellness.

With the knowledge gained from Arnold Ehret, Dr. Robert Young, and Dr. Robert Morse, I significantly improved my health. The only lingering issue was headaches, but they became less frequent and less severe. My journey involved various cleanses, fasts, and a default diet of fruits during the day and a salad with steamed vegetables in the evening. I avoided nuts and seeds and tried not to consume excessive fats. However, there were still a few missing pieces to the puzzle of health that I will explain further in the chapter titled "Natural Hygiene."

What caused my symptoms to worsen during my young adult life?

- Receiving the Hepatitis B vaccine

- Using pharmaceutical drugs like Tylenol 3's, Advil, sleeping pills, and birth control

- Suffering from head/face trauma and a broken collarbone due to two major car accidents

- Poor dietary and lifestyle habits

- Regular and excessive alcohol consumption

- Experiencing traumatic life situations and high levels of stress

The symptoms I suffered from and eventually healed myself from include:

- Chronic fatigue

- Excessive nail biting

- Cysts all over my legs

- Skin rashes and age spots

- Skin tags

- Varicose veins

- Severe depression and negative thoughts

- Poor eyesight

- Substance dependency

- Weekly or daily migraine headaches

- Itchy and dry scalp and skin

- Acne and other skin issues

- Thinning eyebrows

- Alcoholism

- Anger issues

- Poor memory and memory loss

-Loss of motor skills / mobility at random times

Living in pain and discovering which foods to eliminate to alleviate that pain made it easier for me to choose foods that served my health. Pain can be a powerful motivator, and I noticed that most people only make healthier changes when they are suffering.

Although I felt great overall, my healing journey had its ups and downs. I experienced periods of feeling unwell, tired, and irritable as old symptoms resurfaced during the healing process and my body eliminated wastes. I witnessed the elimination of parasites and mucoid plaque from my body, fully aware of the process because I immersed myself in the information. I accepted and embraced the ups and downs as part of the healing process, being grateful for the opportunity to restore my health. Once you experience restored health, it becomes a powerful motivation to continue eating the healthy foods that helped you regain vitality and well-being.

Today, I have a sense of calmness, free from anxiety and pain. My mental clarity has improved in ways I never thought possible. I've regained my ability to dream, and my poor short-term memory has improved. I have transformed into a completely different person. I am grateful to myself, my body, and those who shared their knowledge with me over the past 9 years for this remarkable change.

The best advice I can offer to anyone seeking health and healing is to avoid getting caught up in labels like "raw vegan" or "fruitarian." The key to success lies in establishing a solid foundation by consuming the foods that are natural for us as human beings. When we focus on eating what aligns with our natural design, we don't need a specific "diet." Over time, our health will naturally improve.

Health and disease both develop gradually, so it's important for you to take control of your health. Our daily choices accumulate over the years, and how we feel today reflects our past dietary and lifestyle choices. I hope my story inspires you to take charge of your own health if you haven't already. Ultimately, it all boils down to making consistent, correct dietary / lifestyle choices over a long period of time, allowing the body to heal itself gradually.

Chapter 3
Dr. Robert Young

Dr. Robert Young, an experienced health researcher, author, and American Naturopathic practitioner, is known for promoting an "Alkaline Diet" through his book "The PH Miracle" and is the author of over 50 books. With over 40 years of expertise, Dr. Young has become one of the most famous – and infamous - figures in the medical field, indicating his significant impact. He holds multiple credentials, including a Master of Science in nutrition and a Doctor of Science in Chemistry and Biology. He is a highly sought after keynote speaker at medical conferences around the world and has made multiple guest appearances on a variety of TV and radio programs.

 Dr. Young's focus on the alkaline diet stems from the belief that maintaining a balanced pH is crucial for good health. He emphasizes that an acidic body pH creates an environment for disease and germs to thrive. The core principle of the PH Miracle Diet, as taught by Dr. Young, revolves around maintaining a healthy pH balance in the body. He stresses that an acidic pH creates an environment conducive to disease and pathogens. To achieve optimal health, Dr. Young advocates for an alkaline-rich diet consisting of greens, vegetables, plant fats, and some fish. The recommended ratio is consuming approximately 80% non-acidic foods and 20% acidic foods. Raw, alkaline, plant-based foods, along with ample water and plant fats, are encouraged. Dr. Young suggests moderate consumption of high-carbohydrate vegetables, select grains, and fresh fish. Foods to avoid include meats (excluding fish), dairy products, eggs, alcohol, carbonated drinks, traditional tea, dairy-based smoothies, and fruit juices. While fruits are not promoted, Dr. Young advocates for a variety of supplements, pH drops, juice powders, vitamins, green juices, and salts, among others.

His research, which challenges the "germ theory" and questions mainstream medicine, has been published in reputable journals such as the Journal of Alternative and Complementary Medicine. Dr. Young also emphasizes the harmful effects of vaccines and extensively studies the impact of diet and pharmaceutical substances on blood integrity.

Among the five authors and health advocates I've studied, Dr. Young stands out. Although I don't fully agree with his teachings on diet and health, his book was the first one I read that opened my mind to the possibility of healing and thriving on a plant-based diet without animal products. Dr. Young's information was the first to connect our dietary choices with disease and health issues.

It's worth noting that Dr. Young recommends fish as part of the diet, which I disagree with. Fish, like other meats, is highly putrefactive and protein-rich. Contrary to popular belief, fish isn't a healthier option compared to other meats. It adds an acidic burden to the body due to the breakdown of proteins into amino acids during digestion.

Before diving into Arnold Ehret's "Mucusless Diet Healing System," I initially incorporated Dr. Young's dietary recommendations into my life. It served as my first "transition diet" before discovering Arnold Ehret's teachings. While I quickly shifted to Ehret's approach, I acknowledge the impact of Dr. Young's information in leading me to explore Natural Hygiene and eliminating harmful foods like dairy, eggs, and meat. In fact, it was Dr. Young's book that motivated us to give up our organic farming operation.

Over time, as I embraced Ehret's dietary recommendations, my health issues gradually improved. However, I owe the initial groundwork to Dr. Young's advice, which pushed me to eliminate some of the most detrimental foods from my diet. Although I didn't consume fish frequently, as I strived for self-sufficiency in growing my own food, Arnold Ehret's work later enlightened me about the harmful effects of consuming fish.

I was living on our 7-acre farm when a stranger recommended Dr. Robert Young's book called "The PH Miracle." We were at a seed exchange in Penticton BC, selling and trading local, organic, heirloom seeds we had collected from our plants the previous year. During our conversation, this random lady started discussing our family's health. Although I didn't appear visibly unhealthy, she accurately pointed out that I was suffering from poor health, despite being only 35 years old. She mentioned that we all had candida, and if one family member had it, the others likely did too. It took me some time to understand her statement. Families often have similar eating habits, so if one person suffers, others tend to follow suit. Poor eating habits and disease tend to run in families. This explains why when one family member gets sick, others may appear to "catch" the illness. Sickness and disease are a result of our internal choices rather than contagious factors. The lady at the seed exchange had a natural appearance and a carefree attitude. Her insights into our family's health made a strong impact, especially since I was already seeking answers to my own health issues. Despite making significant changes to my diet and lifestyle, such as moving to an organic farm, I hadn't found the solutions I so desperately sought. At that time, around 80-90% of the food on our plates came from our farm, a significant achievement compared to our previous city life where everything was store-bought. I was known as the "organic queen" among family and friends, determined to heal and feel better. This insightful lady insisted we read Dr. Robert Young's book, "The PH Miracle," immediately, as it would help us improve our health. It struck me as interesting that she initiated the discussion on health, even though we had never met before the seed exchange.

After the seed exchange, we went to a nearby bookstore and bought Dr. Young's book. We eagerly read it as soon as we got home. The book surprised me because I had always believed that meat, raw milk, and eggs were necessary for good health. I had briefly tried eliminating meat from my diet when I lived in the city, but once we moved to the farm and had to deal with meat daily, I started eating it again. Although I felt good during that time without meat, I couldn't resist the influence of those around me who still consumed it. Moving to the farm, I hoped it would help heal my health issues, but I had never seriously considered a diet without animal products because everyone I knew ate them, and I believed they were essential for health. I was unfamiliar with the term "vegan," although I knew about "vegetarianism" from my previous attempt to give up meat in the city. However, my family thought I was strange for avoiding meat, and I became the difficult one during family meals, which led me to abandon the vegetarian diet once we moved to the farm. I joined in eating meat to fit in, especially since we were raising animals for meat on our farm. It was the only time in my life that I questioned the necessity of eating meat. Like most people, I followed family habits and grew up believing that meat and dairy were crucial for a healthy diet. Fortunately, my family didn't consume much meat, mostly ground beef. The first time I had steak was in high school when we split one steak into four portions among my dad, myself, and my two sisters. I watched commercials promoting eggs and milk, and like most people, I believed they were essential for good health. If only I knew then what I know now, I could have spared myself a lot of pain and suffering from childhood into adulthood. Reading Dr. Young's book felt like a revelation, opening a new and exciting world. I was always plagued by a sense of being unhealthy and something being wrong with me. The book gave me hope for a pain-free and happier life, and I was eager to incorporate the newfound knowledge into my life.

After reading Dr. Young's book, we faced a dilemma. We were living on a farm, relying on it for our livelihood, supplying organic meat, eggs, and raw milk to customers and friends who praised us for it. It was scary to think about abandoning the farm and letting go of everything we had built. However, Dr. Young's book had a profound impact on us, giving us hope for an alternative and improved lifestyle. We felt compelled to make a change. It didn't make sense to continue producing and consuming animal meats and products that we now knew were not healthy. Additionally, we had grown tired of the more unpleasant aspects of farming, such as slaughtering and processing animals, finding it cruel, disgusting, and stressful. We made the decision to find suitable homes for all our animals, making sure they wouldn't be used for food. With that assurance, the people were given the animals for free. Now, we no longer needed the 7-acre farm, and we chose to move on. Our focus shifted towards our personal healing, growing fruit trees, gardening, and producing healthy, organic fruits and vegetables.

I can't express enough how much better I felt after following Dr. Young's dietary recommendations. However, it's important to note that feeling better after changing one's diet doesn't automatically mean the diet is correct. Often, people feel better because they've eliminated other unhealthy foods from their diet. In my case, I made a drastic change by immediately cutting out meats, dairy, and eggs. So, the credit for feeling improvements in my health can't solely be attributed to the high-fat intake of avocados and oils recommended by Dr. Young. Looking back, I realize that I felt better because I simplified my diet compared to how I used to eat, which often leads to improved well-being. This aspect is often overlooked. For instance, when someone adopts a predominantly meat-based "Carnivore Diet" and starts feeling better, many would attribute it to the meat. However, what goes unnoticed is that the person has eliminated other harmful foods, simplifying their diet. By reducing the variety of disease-causing foods, some symptoms can be alleviated. However, over time, on a carnivore diet, the heavy consumption of complex, stimulating meats can lead to a decline in well-being. The initial honeymoon period eventually gives way to negative effects as symptoms arise. This phenomenon can be perplexing. Similar patterns can be observed with "Ketogenic" diets, where people feel great in the first year but then experience negative effects from their high-fat intake. It's crucial to understand that these diets are not inherently health-promoting, regardless of how healthy they may seem.

The notion that our thoughts or beliefs can change the effects of our diet is misguided. If we regularly consume suboptimal foods, our poor eating habits will burden our bodies, deplete our energy, and override any positive habits we may have. Any changes made to a non-health-promoting diet only provide temporary relief until symptoms resurface. I've witnessed this pattern countless times over the years. What people believe versus what is true can cause significant harm to ourselves.

I no longer support Dr. Young's dietary recommendations, mainly because he advises people to avoid fruit almost entirely. He categorizes fruit sugar (fructose) with other sugars like processed sugars found in sweets, breads, and beans. Additionally, he promotes excessive consumption of fats from processed plant oils and whole plant fats like avocados. Over time, I've realized that an excessive intake of fats may not be healthy, and it's easy to overdo it. While occasionally including some avocado or whole plant fats is fine, I believe recommending daily consumption of processed oils such as olive oil can lead to health issues.

According to Dr. John McDougall and other plant-based doctors, the consumption of processed oils is a significant factor contributing to the growing epidemic of health problems in the

Western world, including heart disease and diabetes. When I first read Dr. Young's recommendations, I eliminated dairy, eggs, and meat from my diet, but I still included fish (based on what I read in his book) and occasionally consumed whole grains. Fortunately, I had already removed processed foods, junk food, and restaurant meals from my diet long before moving to the farm, so that part wasn't a challenge for me.

The only food I struggled to eliminate was scrambled eggs. I can vividly recall my last plate of scrambled eggs made from our farm-fresh eggs. After reading Dr. Young's book and deciding to eliminate meat, eggs, and dairy, I made a big salad and topped it with four scrambled eggs for my final meal. That was the last time I ate scrambled eggs, as I was determined to prioritize my well-being above all else. I shed a few tears over my last serving of eggs because I knew it was time to permanently remove them from my diet. Today, I am fully aware that my daily consumption of eggs for most of my adult life was a major source of toxicity in my body. Knowing what I know now, I realize that I was slowly harming myself by eating 3-4 scrambled eggs every day.

While living on the farm, I not only consumed cooked eggs but also raw eggs in my afternoon milkshake. It's no wonder that my health rapidly declined during that time and my headaches worsened. I used to believe that eggs were incredibly healthy and that eating them daily, both cooked and raw, was beneficial. I moved to our organic farm to address my health issues and live a healthier life away from the city, only to discover later that I was doing everything wrong. Ironically, I did find a solution to my health problems while on the farm, just not in the way I had initially anticipated or planned.

Reflecting on my experience, I now realize that Dr. Robert Young's recommendations served as a valuable transitional diet away from my farm-based eating habits. They acted as a steppingstone that led me to discover Arnold Ehret's "Mucusless Diet Healing System" shortly after. I followed Dr. Young's dietary recommendations for approximately six months, but fortunately, I didn't incorporate any of his recommended supplements or purchase items from his online store. In hindsight, this turned out to be a blessing because I could have spent a significant amount of money and burdened myself unnecessarily.

I find Dr. Young's dietary advice to be insightful and helpful, particularly his recommendations to eliminate meat, dairy, eggs, and processed foods from the diet while incorporating plenty of greens. However, I disagree with his suggestion to include daily fats like olive oil, coconut oil, or avocados for breakfast. I believe that during the body's elimination mode from 4 am to 12 pm, it's best to break the fast with water-rich, hydrating simple foods such as fruits or a glass of water.

After a couple of months of following Dr. Young's dietary recommendations, I began to experience some relief from my symptoms. During that period, I included olive oil, whole grains, and occasional fish meals in my diet. These additions helped me avoid missing or craving the other foods like meats, eggs, and dairy that I had recently eliminated. This is why I believe Dr. Young's diet served as a beneficial transition, helping me bridge the gap between my old dietary habits and the new ones that would become a permanent part of my life.

According to Dr. Robert Morse, Dr. John McDougall, and Arnold Ehret, fats slow down digestion, contribute to mucus formation within the body, and can lead to weight gain. From my own experience and experiments, I have found that including daily fats in the diet does not promote health. In fact, I felt better when I eliminated fats from my diet for 120 consecutive days while being mindful of keeping my fat intake low (10% of daily dietary intake).

After reading Arnold Ehret's information and striving to follow a "Mucusless diet" for healing purposes, I didn't include fats in my diet for years, except for naturally occurring fats in fruits, vegetables, and greens. However, during that time, I was still healing and had lingering waste from my past dietary habits, so the effects of certain foods on my body weren't as obvious. Now, more than nine years after reading Dr. Young's book, and having successfully healed my health issues, I am more attuned to how foods affect my body, and I avoid those that don't serve me.

Dr. Young advises against consuming fruits, but I strongly disagree with this recommendation. In my experience, a diet that includes 50-70% fruit daily is vital for maintaining good health. While I acknowledge Dr. Young's expertise in studying blood and his extensive credentials, I believe he may be misinterpreting the effects of fruit consumption on blood.

It's possible that the subjects Dr. Young tests his theories on are already unhealthy to begin with, which could influence his conclusions. It's important to consider that the standards of health can vary in today's world, and what is considered "healthy" may not reflect the benefits of a fruit-based diet. Many conventional blood tests use a subjective definition of health based on the average population, which may not apply to individuals consuming a high fruit diet. Additionally, blood tests are only a reflection of that particular moment in time which does not reflect overall health.

After listening to several of Dr. Young's lectures, I have come to the tentative conclusion that he doesn't believe fruits promote health due to the way they affect blood composition. However, I wonder if his interpretation overlooks the cleansing and hydrating effects of fruits, which could be mistaken as negative. It's worth noting that there are other raw foodists who share similar views on fruit, emphasizing the importance of greens and vegetables instead. But from my perspective, fruits are easily digested, visually appealing, delicious, hydrating, and packed with essential vitamins, fiber, and minerals.

Dr. Young's recommended breakfast of steamed broccoli with avocado, for example, is not as appetizing compared to a fresh serving of raw fruit. While Dr. John McDougall also advises limited fruit intake, at least he acknowledges that fruits are part of a healthy diet and recognizes them as whole foods. It's truly perplexing when someone claims that fruits are unhealthy, as if they believe nature itself made an error.

Based on my own research, experience, and acquired knowledge, I firmly believe that eliminating fruits from the diet eliminates the opportunity to build a healthy, disease-free body. Humans are naturally frugivores, and our cells require fructose (fruit sugar) for optimal functioning. Fruits, with their simple sugars (fructose), enter cells easily and provide proper cellular fuel. Fructose doesn't rely on insulin as a carrier for absorption into cells for energy. Moreover, a high fruit diet can help hydrate and break up hardened mucus and waste, while also neutralizing acidity. This contradicts Dr. Young's perspective on fruits, as he believes they are not alkaline and should be avoided.

To gain a comprehensive understanding of why Dr. Young

believes fruits are not health-promoting, I recommend visiting his website or reading his book. It's important to study both sides of the argument to have a balanced perspective. Dr. Young conducted microscopic analyses of human blood before and after fruit consumption, leading him to conclude that fruits do not contribute to healthy blood.

I also disagree with Dr. Young's recommendations regarding supplements and vitamins. He offers a wide range of products on his website, but personally, I wouldn't take any of them. From my studies of experts like Dr. Robert Morse, Arnold Ehret, Natural Hygiene, and even Dr. John McDougall, I've learned that supplements and vitamins can disrupt the body's natural balance and contribute to waste buildup. If a substance is not a whole food in its natural form, it's not inherently health-promoting or usable by the body.

Fortunately, I have always trusted my intuition and avoided supplements and vitamins for the most part throughout my life. It doesn't make sense to me that good health would rely on man-made products indefinitely, suggesting that we cannot achieve health without them.

One common argument for taking supplements is that our food and soil are depleted. However, it's important to recognize that if our soil is depleted, everything that follows will also be depleted. Healthy plants cannot grow or thrive in depleted conditions. Over the years, I've observed that many individuals feel the need to take something for their health, as if it's not enough to solely focus on improving their lifestyle. Simplicity is a foreign concept in the field of health and healing, even though it is the path that truly helps rebuild our well-being.

While reading Herbert Shelton's book "Human Life, It's Philosophy and Laws," I came across an interesting story about a doctor. This doctor noticed that patients who didn't take any herbs or medicines for their ailments recovered faster than those who did. To test his theory, the doctor offered his patients tinctures that were just water, but he presented them as medicine. That's called the Placebo Effect. Surprisingly, the patients who believed they were taking something experienced significant healing and recovered more quickly than those who suppressed their body's natural healing ability by taking actual substances. The powers of the human mind and body when allowed to function in their natural states are amazing.

 Sometimes, I wish I had something specific to recommend for people to take, but there is very little I can sell or suggest apart from making proper dietary and lifestyle choices. The body's ability to heal itself is not dependent on taking external substances; it is the body itself that possesses the true healing power. However, for the body to heal, we must create the right conditions by acquiring proper knowledge and allowing the body to do its job. We need to get out of our own way and understand that less is often more. This is a principle I frequently emphasize.

 During the initial stages of my health journey, I incorporated much of Dr. Young's information for around six months before transitioning to Arnold Ehret's recommendations. I cannot disregard the role Dr. Young's information played in my journey; therefore, I must dedicate this chapter to him as I continue my quest for the truth about our species' appropriate dietary requirements.

In summary, Dr. Young's contributions revolve around advocating for an alkaline diet to maintain pH balance for overall health. He combines his expertise in nutrition, research, and microscopy to shed light on the importance of dietary choices and their impact on our health.   Although I no longer follow Dr. Young's recommendations, I still occasionally listen to his lectures and read his research, particularly on the topic of "blood." This is because I'm conducting my own research on RH- blood types, which I intend to research further. Dr. Young offers unique insights and approaches, demonstrating his ability to think outside the box.

I won't include Dr. Robert Young's teachings and recommendations in later chapters because his teachings diverge significantly from those of Professor Arnold Ehret, Dr. Robert Morse, Dr. John McDougall, Dr. Joel Fuhrman, and Natural Hygiene, which I consider to be more accurate. While Dr. Young offers some helpful information, he also promotes harmful practices such as daily consumption of processed oils, vitamins, and fish. However, I don't dismiss him entirely, and I encourage you to explore his information on your own. He has appeared in Harvard Lectures on YouTube and has some informative content on his website.

You can find out more about Dr. Robert Young at <u>www.</u>
<u>drrobertyoung.com</u>

Chapter 4
<u>Who Was Professor Arnold Ehret?</u>

Professor Arnold Ehret was a renowned health educator and advocate for natural healing. Born on July 29, 1866, in Germany, Ehret dedicated his life to understanding the human body's potential for optimal health through fasting, proper diet and lifestyle choices.

Ehret's journey towards health and wellness began after experiencing his own health challenges. At the age of 31, Arnold Ehret was diagnosed with "Bright's Disease," a kidney inflammation. This led him to explore natural healing methods. He visited sanitariums and countless doctors. Ehret eventually decided to stop eating as a last-ditch effort for his health. Surprisingly, approximately a week later, he found that he felt better and had more vitality and strength than ever before. This unintentional fasting experience led him to gain firsthand knowledge of the body's healing capabilities through fasting.

In his pursuit of healing, Ehret discovered the power of fasting and cleansing the body from accumulated toxins. This revelation led him to develop his revolutionary system, known as the Mucusless Diet Healing System. Ehret believed that mucus-forming foods were responsible for most disease issues and advocated for a proper transition diet consisting of primarily mucusless foods.

Ehret's insights and teachings gained widespread attention and acclaim, and he became a highly sought-after lecturer and author. His most notable works include "The Mucusless Diet Healing System" and "Rational Fasting," which continue to inspire and guide individuals seeking natural healing and improved well-being.

Throughout his life, Ehret emphasized the importance of

understanding and respecting the body's innate wisdom. He believed that by adopting a mucus-free diet and incorporating fasting as a regular practice, individuals could restore their health, vitality, and longevity.

Sadly, Professor Arnold Ehret died at the young age of 56. On October 9, 1922, Arnold Ehret, at the height of his career, tragically passed away in what was reported as a sudden and unfortunate accident. According to accounts, he suffered a basal fracture of the skull, leading to instant death. The incident occurred on a dark and foggy night, with the sidewalk being described as "oil soaked" and unusually slippery. Ehret slipped and fell backward on an oil-soaked driveway, landing with significant force on the back of his head, resulting in the fatal injury. He was pronounced dead on arrival at the hospital.

This incident took place shortly after one of Ehret's highly sought-after and sold-out lectures, where attendees paid a hefty fee, equivalent to around $1300 in today's value, to benefit from his knowledge and insights on health and healing. Ehret's popularity was on the rise as his advice and methods were reportedly helping people improve their well-being. Some people believe that his untimely death was not an accident, attributing it to a deliberate act. There is limited information available about the incident, and unfortunately, Ehret's passing cut short what many believed was a promising career. It is speculated that his success and potential impact on the pharmaceutical industry might have made him a perceived threat. Despite the lack of documentation on the incident, Ehret's early death was a significant loss, as many feel he had much more to contribute in the field of health and healing. His legacy lives on as a source of inspiration for those who strive for optimal health and well-being.

Ehret was a true pioneer of his time, and he introduced the concept of "Mucusless" foods to describe a dietary approach that minimizes the accumulation of mucus within the body, which he believed to be a contributing factor to disease. Today, despite his teachings, the majority of people still consume "Mucus Forming Foods," which can be observed in the increasing numbers of disease diagnoses each year.

Arnold Ehret's remarkable journey and his ability to heal himself and assist others have left a lasting impact on the field of health and wellness. His insights and teachings continue to resonate with those seeking alternative approaches to health and the prevention of disease.

Arnold Ehret's teachings centered on the concept that all diseases stem from a single source, which is internal toxicity within the body. According to his philosophy, the various disease names assigned to specific sets of symptoms only serve to confuse people and divert them from understanding the fundamental truth – that there is ultimately only "One Disease" and one underlying cause for all illnesses.

Given the importance of Ehret's teachings, it is recommended that anyone interested in enhancing their well-being or seeking to heal their health problems should consider reading these two books. It is worth noting that as time passes, these books may become less readily available, so it is advisable to obtain them before they become scarce. By delving into Ehret's writings, individuals can gain valuable insights into his philosophy and potentially discover approaches to better health and healing.

Many individuals discover Arnold Ehret's teachings and the Mucusless Diet Healing System only after exhausting other options and realizing the limitations of the medical system. It's unfortunate that more people are not aware of the simplicity and effectiveness of his information, which can help individuals heal themselves without resorting to costly drugs or procedures. Ehret's books are affordable, packed with life-saving information, and relatively short reads. It's surprising how many people claim to understand Ehret's recommendations without actually reading his books. To truly grasp his system and avoid misconceptions, thorough reading is essential.

To begin the healing process, we must be willing to let go of our unhealthy habits and choices that led to our health issues. It can be hard for individuals to accept that their diet and lifestyle may be making them sick, and they may be resistant to trying healthier alternatives. Letting go of restaurant and fast foods completely is often a difficult step that many people are unwilling to take. Even in "Raw Vegan" or "Vegan" restaurants, preparations may include harmful ingredients such as toxic salts, oils, processed vegan foods, nutritional yeast, and sugar. Taking control of our own meals is the first step toward rebuilding our health.

 It's important to acknowledge that the process of transitioning to a healthy diet and lifestyle involves trial and error. Changing everything overnight is not realistic, as nature works gradually, and overwhelming oneself with too many changes at once can be counterproductive. Once we learn the truth about health, it's crucial not to lose sight of it. True healing requires a willingness, dedication, and long-term commitment to healthier choices. Undoing the effects of a lifetime of unhealthy habits takes time.

Healing is not always easy; individuals will face tests and temptations along the way. However, learning Arnold Ehret's information can save time and provide clarity amidst the confusion. Becoming our own doctor is crucial, as no one knows us better than ourselves, and no one can do the healing for us. The Mucusless Diet Healing System's principles go beyond simply knowing which foods are "Mucusless" or "Mucus Forming." It is recommended to read Ehret's literature to fully understand his teachings, as no one explains it as well as he does.

Learning to recognize when the body is eliminating waste and understanding how to navigate through these eliminations without excessive worry about symptoms is an important aspect of Ehret's teachings. He also covers topics such as food combinations and fasting. Proper fasting requires understanding when to fast, how long to fast, and most importantly, how to break a fast based on individual health conditions. The transition period will vary for each person based on their current health, motivation, and circumstances.

In all honesty, "The Mucusless Diet Healing System" is not overly complicated to learn, and it makes sense. After reading it, I was shocked by its simplicity and its potential for healing and maintaining good health. I was willing to put in the necessary dietary work for a pain-free existence. The most challenging aspect for many people is committing to a long-term lifestyle rather than viewing it as just a temporary diet. It's crucial to understand that it's not just about learning which foods to eat or avoid for health. It requires comprehension of what occurs within the body, such as recognizing uncomfortable elimination symptoms, which may deter individuals and cause them to mistake the body's healing efforts for new health problems.

This misunderstanding may lead them to give up and seek alternative solutions. That's why reading the book is so important, yet it's surprising how many people adamantly choose not to do so.

I often wondered why Dr. Morse didn't include the "Mucusless Diet Healing System" as a proper transition diet in his teachings, especially considering that he read Arnold Ehret's work. Dr. Morse mentioned being inspired by Ehret's book in the 60s, which led him to undertake a six-month orange fast/cleanse to heal his own health issues. While I understand that Ehret's system is challenging to explain and that his books provide the best explanation, I believe it's somewhat irresponsible to overlook the importance of a transition diet.

Sadly, most people are looking for quick fixes or easy-to-follow information that requires minimal learning. I'm not saying that Ehret's system is difficult to follow or understand, but it does require a deeper understanding beyond just eating fruit only for healing, which is what Dr. Morse teaches. I believe Dr. Morse may have felt the need to simplify the dietary aspect of his protocols because his patients are very ill and do not have time to "mess around", but in doing so, he omitted the transition diet which can be extremely beneficial for the individuals that are not dealing with chronic disease. I will note that Dr. Morse includes the *Mucusless Diet* and *Rational Fasting* as "further reading" in the bibliography at the end of his *Sourcebook*. And as Prof. Spira brought to my attention, Dr. Morse also sold copies of the *Mucusless Diet and Rational Fasting* for years in his clinic's store. In Dr. Morses *Detox Miracle Sourcebook* he also mentions that there is a place for cooked vegetables when needed. Teaching people to only eat fruit, berries, and melons is a protocol for individuals with serious disease issues, but it's not practical for the average person wanting to improve their health because it often leads to individuals struggling to stick to a fruit-only diet. When cravings inevitably arise, they may turn to less-than-ideal foods, which may not have been the case if a proper transition had been incorporated.

If individuals learned the principles of the Mucusless Diet Healing System and understood why transitioning is vital for building long-lasting, sustainable healthy habits, they would find it easier to deal with cravings and satiation. After reading and learning the system, someone struggling with cravings could navigate such situations more effectively. Instead of turning to their familiar harmful foods, they might choose to bake a squash and pair it with a leafy green salad, for example. And if the craving persisted, they would have learned other less harmful options to turn to instead of reverting to old habits.

The idea is to satisfy cravings with foods that are significantly less harmful to our overall health than the actual craved food, but we need to read the book to learn what those foods are.

It's easy to overlook or disbelieve the fact that our past dietary habits and lifestyle choices led to the development of our health issues because symptoms often appear out of nowhere. I've heard countless times, "He/she was perfectly healthy until suddenly diagnosed with cancer." Some people believe that a diagnosis comes suddenly and out of the blue. However, nothing is truly sudden. Cancer has been building and developing within the body for 10, 20, 30+ years. It's just that by the time we realize it, the symptoms have progressed to a noticeable and undeniable point.

We live in a world where people seek fast results and quick fixes. People are often unwilling to invest years of time and energy in carefully following a dietary system that requires individual thought and application. It's much easier to pay someone to design a meal plan or dictate how to live and eat. What most people don't want to do is become their own doctor because it feels scary and unfamiliar. However, when we've exhausted every other avenue, it becomes essential to become our own doctor, especially for the purpose of self-healing.

When we learn Arnold Ehret's information, we realize why a standardized meal plan simply won't work. Healing isn't a straightforward path; our habits and routines change as we progress and adapt to our healing journey. We must learn to listen to our bodies so that we can make subtle adjustments within our own routines. Arnold Ehret warned against immediately transitioning from a standard diet to an all-fruit diet without a proper transition, as it may not effectively cleanse the body from years of accumulated waste and could even be dangerous in some cases. A systematic approach is necessary to cleanse the body from decades of accumulated filth and waste matter.

Truth be told, we don't have to achieve a perfect cleanse to experience relief from our unwanted symptoms. Even if we're not eliminating all the old, stored-up waste from within, we can still find tremendous relief by eliminating the most burdensome foods from our diet.

When the body finally receives adequate digestive rest from foods that burden the digestive system, it often redirects freed-up energy towards elimination and healing.

There's one aspect where Arnold Ehret excelled above others, and that is in interpreting the healing process within the body. The misinterpretation of symptoms has led most doctors and healthcare professionals to offer harmful health advice, as they label each separate symptom expressed by the body (stemming from one root cause) as a separate disease. The individual labeling of symptoms as separate diseases only serves to confuse everyone involved, with the only beneficiaries being the pharmaceutical companies who can create separate drugs for each symptom.

In my opinion, the misinterpretation of all things lies at the core of many issues we face in the world today. Interpretation shapes our understanding, and if we fail to interpret or comprehend nature and its workings accurately, the consequences can be disastrous.

When I delved into the realm of health, I found Arnold Ehret's book to be the most significant and impactful one I have come across thus far. Reading his books provided me with a clear understanding of the root causes of disease and how we can rebuild our health. The story of how I stumbled upon Ehret's book, "Rational Fasting," is quite remarkable, and I believe it's worth sharing.

I was enjoying a beautiful afternoon on the shared land where I lived. Upstairs in one of the outbuildings, there was a cozy space for relaxation that was open to everyone. Sasha, who also resided on the property, had some of her books and personal belongings in the room. Curiosity got the better of me, and I found myself browsing through her bookshelf. Among the titles, Arnold Ehret's book, "Rational Fasting," immediately caught my attention. It's important to note that at that time, I had never heard of Arnold

Ehret or had any prior knowledge about fasting. Nevertheless, I decided to borrow the book and explore its contents.

As I made my way downstairs with Arnold Ehret's book in hand, my father dropped by for an unexpected visit. He was heading up the stairs just as I was going down, and we crossed paths midway. When he noticed the book in my hands, I distinctly remember his words from over 9 years ago. He exclaimed, "Oh, that guy? He just irks me!" My father asked if I intended to read the book, and then he made a comment about Arnold Ehret being a "show off" with his knee bends. It felt as though he was trying to put me off from reading it (which I later realized why he might have done so). He asked me to share my thoughts on the book after I finished reading it. Once he left, I started reading, beginning my journey with Arnold Ehret's work.

A few days after the conversation on the stairs, I had to call my dad. Having finished reading Arnold Ehret's book, I couldn't contain my excitement. I told my dad that this was the most significant book I had come across in my entire life! I was captivated by Ehret's words, and the impact of his ideas resonated deeply within me.

 As I turned each page, I was astounded by the profound insights and revelations contained within. The simplicity of our diet and lifestyle for achieving optimal health became abundantly clear. It was a revelation that had never crossed my mind before: the complex mixtures of food we consume, often containing numerous ingredients, greatly contribute to the health issues that plague so many individuals today.

I found myself unable to put Ehret's book down, immersed in its pages and hungry for more knowledge. The clarity and simplicity of his teachings were truly remarkable, and I felt a renewed sense of purpose and direction in my own journey toward better health.

Later, I began to understand why I felt that my father unintentionally discouraged me from reading Arnold Ehret's book. It's interesting because when we were standing on the stairs that afternoon and he made those comments about the book, I had a fleeting moment of doubt. I briefly considered running back upstairs to return the book, but thankfully, I didn't.

At 19, my father embarked on a solitary journey, without the support of like-minded individuals, as this was before the internet and social media connected people. He faced a lack of understanding from his family to the point where they considered committing him. Seeking sunshine and fruit, he moved to Hawaii to practice the Mucusless Diet Healing System. Although I don't know why he eventually deviated from it, I've witnessed others lose sight of the truth, and I refuse to let that happen to me. I was born seven years after he abandoned the diet, but it feels as if this knowledge is in my blood—like fruit sugar coursing through my veins.

When I called my father a few days later to tell him how significant the book was to me, he responded with, "Let's see how you are in a few years." He understood that real knowledge and experience on diet and lifestyle take time to develop.

It's worth mentioning that my father lived an hour's drive away, and his unannounced visit was quite rare. The timing of his visit that day, coinciding with me holding the very book that would later transform my life, was quite remarkable. What were the chances?

When we make healthier changes to our lifestyle and diet, it often clashes with the habits and choices of those around us. Most people resist change and struggle to understand dietary choices that seem unconventional to them. When we no longer share the same food preferences with our family and friends, they may perceive it as a personal rejection. Witnessing healthier choices forces them to reflect on their own lifestyle and eating habits, which many people find uncomfortable and prefer to avoid. People tend to follow the path of least resistance.

Incorporating healthier changes is often seen as extreme or crazy by others who don't comprehend the reasons behind it. Some may even attack you for your choices because they find your new habits so outlandish. From my perspective, our physical well-being is directly influenced by the food we consume. The nutrients we choose to ingest shape our bodies over time. When we reject commonly shared foods, family members and friends may take it personally, viewing us as outsiders. They may lash out because they cannot understand why we would abandon the foods we once enjoyed together.

Radical changes in diet can provoke strong reactions from others who may resist sudden shifts, especially if they didn't initiate them. People may reject our efforts rather than evaluate their value, finding it easier to reject us instead. If we can't effectively explain and have others accept our choices, stress and misunderstandings can arise. I encourage individuals to understand the information themselves, so they can educate others about their health goals. Writing this book serves as a resource to help others comprehend the improvements they seek in health and quality of life.

One of the most challenging aspects during the body's elimination of stored waste is the inevitable weight and waste loss. Almost everyone (unless already underweight) experiences weight loss when adopting this lifestyle, as it is a necessary part of the healing process. When we eliminate disease- and mucus-forming foods from our diet and focus on a predominantly mucusless, health-promoting diet, the body begins to eliminate years of internal waste. This may result in a temporary "skinny phase" that some people fear and dread. Many of us have gone through this phase, and it can be particularly challenging for men compared to women, as societal norms make it more acceptable for women to be thin. Comments and looks can be difficult to handle. It is crucial to have a deep understanding of this process so that we can explain to concerned others that it is temporary, even though it may take time.

Mothers may become worried when they see their children losing "too much weight" and may make comments that express concern or fear. Those who do not understand this natural process the body goes through may use the "skinny phase" as justification to criticize the natural diet and discredit healthy eating habits. They may try to convince individuals to abandon their healthy path and return to the familiar world of comforting, mucus-forming foods. Unfortunately, many people have given up their health endeavors due to pressure from family, friends, and acquaintances who attempt to deter them based on their own fears, opinions, comments, and disapproving looks.

After more than 9 years of incorporating Arnold Ehret's principles into my life, I've learned that it's important to take things slowly. It's not a race but a lifestyle that requires time and mastery. Nature works gradually, and our health follows the same path.

Understanding the Mucusless Diet Healing System helps us build lasting dietary habits and handle cravings and eliminations. In the beginning, I got overly excited and fasted without proper preparation, feeling exhausted and lethargic. To assess your health, try a 3-day water fast or incorporate more raw foods into your diet. I now realize the progress I've made health-wise. Setbacks and cravings are normal, but the system teaches us how to deal with them. Our food choices evolve over time, transitioning to the foods our bodies are designed to eat. Using less harmful options like coconut bread helped me manage cravings during the elimination phase. As we become cleaner, our tastes and desires change, reflecting the seasons and food availability. The Mucusless Diet Healing System guides us in making less harmful choices while transitioning to a natural human diet.

I've learned that fasting and avoiding extremes are essential to avoid harm. Reflecting on my father's experience, I now understand why he may have discouraged me from reading Arnold Ehret's book and embracing the Mucusless Diet. He was trying to protect me from the difficulties and pitfalls he had encountered on his own journey.

I initially learned about fasting from Arnold Ehret's books, later delving deeper into the works of Herbert Shelton and other proponents of the Natural Hygiene movement. Over the years, I've done several short water fasts and a couple of seven-day fasts. Nowadays, I only fast once a year in December, unless my body doesn't feel well. When sick, I instinctively fast, following the example of animals. While Ehret didn't recommend long fasting periods, I plan to do an extended fast of 20-40 days in the future when the conditions are ideal, preferably in a warm climate. Ehret emphasizes the importance of building healthy dietary habits over extended fasting. Proper preparation and breaking the fast with the right foods are crucial, as the re-feeding process is as important as the fast itself. If considering fasting, I recommend reading Ehret's books for more information. Both "Rational Fasting" and "The Mucusless Diet Healing System" provide valuable principles that can improve anyone's health, regardless of their location.

In my experience with health-related groups, those who adopt "The Mucusless Diet Healing System" for health and healing tend to follow one of two paths. They either become health coaches and assist others in their healing journey, or they gradually return to a diet that aligns with societal norms, feeling tired of standing out. After healing, the pain we once experienced becomes a distant memory, and we forget its severity. Discovering Ehret's book saved me from falling into dietary misinformation traps and wasting years searching for healing. This knowledge is not new; it has existed since the beginning of time. However, it seems we have forgotten how to nourish and care for ourselves over time. I've observed a lack of accurate teaching about our natural diet among health advocates. While many versions exist, they often miss crucial information, hindering complete healing. If Arnold Ehret were alive today, I would express my gratitude for sharing his knowledge on health and healing, benefiting both myself and the world.

After a few years of following Ehret's teachings, something peculiar happened. I was at the farmer's market, selling the produce we had grown, when I encountered a stranger. An elderly man struck up a conversation with me at our farm stand. He was talking about an old car he had invented years ago. At some point in the story, he mentioned Arnold Ehret's book, "Rational Fasting." What surprised me was that he claimed that Ehret had been murdered in a hit-and-run accident, with his death intentionally covered up. (It's important to note that I had never discussed Ehret's work or the books I had read with anyone at the farmer's market. Thus, when this stranger randomly brought up Ehret's name and stated that his death was not accidental, but a deliberate act, I was shocked and left pondering. I had previously found Ehret's death suspicious when I read about it years ago, but to have a stranger approach me and claim he was murdered left me in a state of wonder.) After purchasing some vegetables, he left, and I never saw him again. I still don't know what that encounter meant, if anything. It left me contemplating the incident throughout the rest of the day. Quite strange indeed.

That man had no knowledge of my online work, my lifestyle, or the fact that I had read Ehret's books. I learned to only discuss my dietary knowledge if someone else brings it up first. I quickly realized it's best to share this information only with those who actively seek it.

Chapter 5
Dr. Robert Morse, ND: A Pioneer in Natural Healing

When it comes to natural healing, few names hold as much weight as Dr. Robert Morse. With over 30 years of clinical experience as a Naturopathic doctor, healer, and herbalist, he has dedicated his life to guiding and assisting people in their journey to overcome various health conditions. From cancer and diabetes to obesity, infertility, and Multiple Sclerosis, Dr. Morse has helped countless individuals find their path to wellness.

Regarded as one of the greatest healers of our modern world within the Raw Food movement, Dr. Morse stands apart due to his deep understanding of why the body exhibits symptoms of disease. Unlike mainstream medical practices that revolve around the "Germ Theory" narrative and the outdated obsession with viruses, Dr. Morse takes a different approach. He believes that the body has the innate ability to heal itself if given the proper environment, which involves following his recommended dietary, environmental, and herbal protocols. His methods and knowledge do not rely on pharmaceuticals, vitamins, supplements, or quick fixes, which is why he remains relatively unknown in mainstream health circles.

Dr. Morse draws inspiration from the teachings of esteemed figures such as Herbert Shelton, Arnold Ehret, Hilton Hotema, T.C. Fry, and many others from our forgotten and possibly hidden past. His wealth of knowledge stems from his extensive experience running clinics, working in hospital emergency rooms, and owning health food stores. As a degreed Biochemist, master herbalist, iridologist, and Naturopathic doctor, Dr. Morse possesses a well-rounded background that enables him to address health issues from multiple angles.

Like many great healers, Dr. Robert Morse faced his own health challenges in his 20s. Growing up on a dairy farm and adhering to a typical, standard diet, he was plagued by recurring headaches, constipation, and blocked sinuses. These issues prompted him to delve deeper into the world of natural healing, leading him to study the works of renowned pioneers in the field. Inspired by what he learned; Dr. Morse embarked on his own personal health journey.

For approximately four years, Dr. Morse adopted an all-fruit diet, primarily centered around oranges, as a means of promoting health and facilitating healing. During a six-month phase within those four years, he even exclusively consumed oranges while living in his van, a practice known as mono-fruit eating. Through this transformative experience, Dr. Morse found the remedy he sought for his health issues and was inspired to share his knowledge about the healing powers of fruits.

In his book, "The Detox Miracle Sourcebook," Dr. Morse provides a chapter titled "A Personal Journey", where readers can gain insight into the experiences that shaped his path to becoming the influential healer he is today.

Today, Dr. Robert Morse's clinic in Florida is experiencing tremendous success and a high demand for his natural healing methods. However, the bustling clinic also serves as a reflection of the increasing number of individuals seeking alternatives to allopathic approaches, such as drugging and surgery. This demand signifies a growing awareness and desire for natural healing solutions. While Dr. Morse is no longer personally seeing patients after many years of doing so, he remains active in his clinic. He oversees a well-trained staff who ensures the clinic continues to operate smoothly. His primary focus now lies in teaching students his extensive knowledge and methods, enabling them to assist others through his healing and detoxification protocols.

To accommodate the widespread interest in his teachings, Dr. Morse offers Detoxification Specialist certificate programs both online and, in a classroom setting in Florida. Having personally studied Dr. Morse's coursework and obtained a Level 1 Detoxification Specialist certification, I have found it to be an invaluable tool in my work of guiding others towards self-healing.

One of Dr. Robert Morse's most remarkable contributions is his book, "The Detox Miracle Sourcebook." I highly recommend this comprehensive healing guide to anyone interested in learning about health and healing. What sets it apart is Dr. Morse's meticulous attention to detail, backed by scientific evidence, as he proves that humans are naturally frugivorous beings. He delves into the detrimental effects of protein and high-protein diets on human health. Furthermore, the book provides valuable insights into what to expect during the body's detoxification process, ensuring readers have a clear understanding and are prepared for the journey ahead.

One quote from Dr. Morse has resonated with me profoundly: *"There are no incurable diseases, just incurable people"*. This statement holds great truth. Over the years, I have encountered numerous individuals who, despite seeking guidance, are unwilling to relinquish the very foods and lifestyle choices that have led to their sickness. They are unwilling to address the root causes and therefore unwilling to commit to the healing process. It saddens me to witness their suffering due to their resistance to change. However, it is crucial to recognize that as individuals make the effort to clean up their diets and lifestyle habits, which contribute to their ailments, their taste buds undergo a transformation. Over time, the foods they initially found unappealing become delicious and satisfying. Achieving true healing requires effort, knowledge, and dedication. While the rewards of restoring one's health are immense, there are no shortcuts or quick fixes. Consequently, my first question to those seeking guidance is always, "Are you willing to give up the foods and substances that have made you sick?" If the answer is no, it is clear they are not yet prepared to embark on the path of reclaiming their well-being.

At the core of Dr. Robert Morse's teachings lies the principle of simplicity in healing. He emphasizes the consumption of whole, unprocessed foods, particularly juicy fruits, berries, and melons. These foods do not burden the digestive system and allow the body to focus its energy on healing. According to Dr. Morse, fruits are hydrating, promote waste elimination, and provide quick and abundant nutrition, making them the optimal food for human health.

Dr. Morse advocates for a predominantly raw food diet, with a strong emphasis on fruit consumption. This approach helps create the ideal internal environment for the body to heal itself by addressing the acidic and toxic wastes that accumulate in the lymphatic system—a primary root cause of various diseases. <u>Like the teachings of Arnold Ehret, Dr. Morse highlights that humans suffer from one disease—internal toxicity—with a multitude of symptoms that tend to overshadow the underlying cause.</u>

For many individuals, the most challenging aspect of Dr. Morse's teachings is the long-term commitment to consuming primarily fruits or simple, whole, raw foods for the duration necessary to facilitate healing. Depending on the individual, this healing process can extend beyond a year or even several years, allowing for the regeneration of damaged tissues, organs, and glands. Dr. Robert Morse sheds light on the importance of "Kidney Filtration" and the crucial role played by the lymphatic system in the healing journey. Understanding these concepts helps individuals grasp the overall process and its significance.

By adopting a diet centered around raw fruits and incorporating simple, whole, raw foods, individuals can provide their bodies with the healthiest, most hydrating, vitamin- and nutrient-rich sustenance available. As the habit of including raw fruit or raw foods in the diet becomes established, the body gradually embarks on its healing journey. However, it is important to remember that healing times cannot be predicted or rushed. They vary for each person and depend on factors such as age, environment, disease stage, genetics, willingness to change, and more.

Dr. Morse also integrates the practice of Iridology into his work, utilizing it as a diagnostic tool to identify obstructions and weaknesses within the body. Through Iridology, he can assess whether an individual will be a slow, moderate, or fast healer based on their unique constitution, which is revealed through the iris. The eyes serve as a mirror or map of our internal condition. For a deeper understanding of Iridology, it is worth exploring the work of Bernard Jensen, as Dr. Morse learned his Iridology knowledge from studying Dr. Jensen's contributions. I, too, have studied Bernard Jensen's work and Dr. Morse's insights into Iridology, finding the knowledge fascinating and enlightening.

When I first encountered Dr. Robert Morse's teachings, I was already immersed in studying Arnold Ehret's "Mucusless Diet Healing System" to address my own health issues. At that time,

I had some reservations about Dr. Morse due to his emphasis on spirituality, which didn't resonate with me. I formed a quick judgment and chose not to explore his health-related information further. I had a personal rule that I would only take health advice from individuals who had achieved the results I desired for myself. I felt that Dr. Morse didn't radiate optimal health, and his extensive discussions on spirituality overshadowed his health teachings. I believed that if he didn't follow his own dietary advice, he couldn't be taken seriously as a teacher.

Looking back, I realize that I failed to consider that many individuals, including Dr. Morse, come from backgrounds of poor health. It is often those who have suffered the most who delve deep into the realm of health and seek to share their knowledge. Additionally, not everyone can outwardly appear in perfect health, especially when they have chosen a path of healing that challenges societal norms. Critics often ask why raw vegans or fruitarians appear unhealthy or sickly. The truth is that individuals who pursue alternative diets may not fit conventional ideas of health, but their dedication stems from their personal journey and the quest for healing. Moreover, timing plays a significant role. When I first encountered Dr. Morse, it simply wasn't the right time for me to benefit from his teachings.

A few years later, a video by Dr. Morse caught my attention, and I decided to listen to what he had to say. His sincerity and honesty resonated with me, and I found him to be down-to-earth. Despite his admission of deviating from a strict fruitarian diet due to personal preferences and circumstances, I valued his honesty. While it's an individual choice whether or not to follow our own dietary advice exactly, I believe that if we present ourselves as teachers, it is important to exemplify the principles we teach. Leading by example is crucial. However, compassion and understanding are also necessary, as everyone has their own choices and limitations. Not everyone can adhere to a species-appropriate diet long-term for various reasons, and as long as they are honest and not pretending otherwise, that is acceptable. I recall Arnold Ehret stating that his personal choices did not change the truth he shared. Nevertheless, as teachers of dietary truths, I believe it is important to do our best to practice what we preach.

Another aspect to consider is experimentation. Although I understand through experience and study that a raw diet consisting of fruits, greens, and vegetables is optimal for our species, I once embarked on a 72-day trial of Dr. John McDougall's "Starch Solution Diet" to gain personal experience and knowledge to speak about his plant-based dietary approach.

After studying and practicing the Mucusless Diet Healing System for several years, I felt it was time to explore Dr. Robert Morse's teachings. I started listening to his YouTube videos on health and detoxification. In just one video, I became captivated by his knowledge and presentation style. To my surprise, Dr. Morse's dietary information proved extremely valuable for healing various disease issues. However, I learned to skip past his discussions on spirituality, focusing solely on the health-related aspects. Unfortunately, I often hesitated to recommend Dr. Morse's information to some individuals due to their dismissal of him as a "quack" when they hear him speak about his spiritual views. While I may not resonate with his spiritual talks, I can accept that those are his own beliefs, allowing me to separate them from his health teachings.

I have observed that important information often appears in our lives when we are ready to receive it. After a few years on the Mucusless Diet Healing System, my health seemed to plateau, and I felt the need to improve my routine and make dietary adjustments instinctively. Continuous improvement and forward progress are core principles of the Mucusless Diet Healing System. The timing of studying Dr. Morse's information seemed perfect for me at that point, as it provided the motivation to delve deeper and embark on detoxification after laying a foundation for it over the past two years.

I must note that today, I no longer view health and healing solely through the lens of detoxification. The term itself implies that we are in control of the healing process and that we must do something different to force the body into a healing state, beyond living in a healthful manner. Here is an article that I recently wrote for our "Monthly Terrain Model Diet Support Group" which I posted on my Applediaries website, which provides further clarification on my evolving perspective.

What is Detox?

Detoxification, from a Terrain Model standpoint, is a natural function carried out by the body to eliminate toxins and waste through its various elimination channels. These eliminative channels include the skin, bowels, urine, breath, uterus, ears, and more, depending on an individual's state of health.

Contrary to popular belief, detoxification is not something we can control or force upon the body using specific substances or interventions. The body is continuously engaged in the process of cleaning and detoxifying itself to the best of its ability.

Heavier detoxification periods, characterized by detoxification symptoms, may occur when the body has enough nerve energy to initiate a cleaning event. This typically happens when the burden on the body is reduced through healthier diet and lifestyle choices, allowing the body to focus on self-healing.

When the body is no longer overwhelmed by frequent heavy digestive periods, it can redirect vital energy toward cleaning itself by eliminating excess internal waste. This can result in detoxification symptoms such as cold and flu-like symptoms.

It is important to differentiate between the body eliminating newly created wastes and the body trying to keep up with waste accumulation from an unnatural diet. By examining our current diet and lifestyle choices, we can gain insights into the body's detoxification process.

If we have been following a clean diet of raw fruits, greens, and vegetables that do not burden the digestive system, it is safe to assume that the body is detoxifying itself from past waste accumulation because we are no longer ingesting unnatural foods that contribute to these waste deposits.

Returning to a natural diet of fruits, greens, and raw foods does not detoxify the body directly. Rather, the body detoxifies itself because the correct conditions are in place for healing to occur.

However, if we regularly consume foods that burden the body, such as mucus- and acid-forming foods, and subsequently experience detoxification symptoms, it indicates that the body is overburdened and struggling to eliminate the excess waste associated with the current diet.

It is worth noting that exposure to toxic chemicals, sprays, and substances can also trigger a detoxification or cleaning event in the body if it has sufficient nerve energy. If the body lacks the necessary energy, these toxins can accumulate and contribute to more serious conditions.

Unfortunately, some individuals in health and healing groups may unknowingly ingest harmful substances such as herbal tinctures, supplements, or vitamins in an attempt to force their bodies into healing or detoxification. However, the body is simply trying to eliminate the excess poisonous waste associated with these substances.

The only safe and natural way to truly cleanse the body is to create the correct conditions for health. This involves returning to a natural diet and allowing the body to heal and correct itself over time, recognizing that the timeframe for healing varies for each person based on factors such as age, past diet, and internal health condition.

By providing the body with the right conditions, we allow the intelligent body to do the rest. It is crucial to get out of the way and practice "Doing Nothing Intelligently" by allowing the body's natural healing processes to unfold. Health is the result of healthy living and creating an environment conducive to self-healing.

Here's a passage from Dr Morse's "Detox Miracle Sourcebook" explaining the detoxification process in his own words:

"It is not uncommon to experience many side effects during detoxification. These include cold and flu-like symptoms, changes in bowel movements, pains of various types, fevers, heartburn, lung congestion, energy loss, swelling and itching, and even vomiting. In this section we will examine each of these possible side effects. Sometimes we will suggest ways to help the cleansing process along, or ways to alleviate the discomfort of this 'healing crisis' as it is called. In general, we encourage you to continue through these side effects in the direction of regeneration.

As the body begins to clean its lymphatic system, the sinus cavities, lungs and most other body tissues will become active in the cleansing process. Do not stop this natural process. This is the only true way to increase the function of your cells and to start your body on the path to regeneration.

You will begin to see a lot of mucus being discharged from the body. This mucus can be clear, yellow, green, and even brown or black. Occasionally you might find blood in the mucus. Don't panic. This blood has been there a while. Congestion is acidic and can cause inflammation and bleeding of tissue. The throat can get very sore. This is just mucus and toxins in the tissues trying to get out. It is best not to use cough drops." – Dr. Robert Morse

Members of the health community often criticize the concept of detoxification, claiming everything can be attributed to detox. In a sense this is true, because the body expresses symptoms as a curative process so our unwanted symptoms can be attributed to the body's natural process of healing. The body is constantly working to maintain homeostasis, or balance, and when it becomes sick, it is a sign that the body is attempting to heal and correct itself.

When the body is not functioning optimally and expressing symptoms, there are generally two reasons for it: either it is undergoing detoxification or dealing with a degenerative condition. In a state of good health, the body experiences continuous balance, but when our diet and lifestyle choices disrupt this balance, it can lead to disease issues that may progress into degenerative conditions if not addressed.

The symptoms we experience are the body's attempts at healing and cleansing itself. By examining our dietary and lifestyle choices, we can discern whether the symptoms are the result of detoxification or the progression of a degenerative condition.

When we lift the burden on the body by adopting a healthy raw diet of fruits and greens, the body can heal itself because vital nerve energy is no longer expended heavily on the complex task of digestion. Fruits and greens are easily digestible and require minimal energy for digestion while supplying the body with all its nutritional needs.

All disease issues stem from an over acidic, waste-filled internal terrain, known as internal toxemia. When the body becomes overwhelmed and experiences waste overload, it may initiate a healing event, often characterized by detoxification symptoms such as cold and flu-like symptoms.

It's important not to focus on individual symptoms that arise during the healing process. If the root causes (diet and lifestyle) have been addressed, the body will heal itself.

There's no need to fear detoxification. Instead, it should be seen as an opportunity to celebrate and rest. During a cleaning event, the body requires nerve energy to carry out its healing processes. Resting and drinking plenty of water allow the body to undergo its healing processes without interference.

Herbert Shelton's quote, *"Life should be built on the conservation of energy"*, emphasizes the importance of conserving energy for the body's healing processes.

While Dr. Robert Morse teaches an all-fruit/raw diet, it is not necessary to jump into such an extreme diet. From a Natural Hygiene perspective, fresh raw fruits should make up about 50% of the diet, while the other 50% should come from leafy greens, tender leaves, and some fats from nuts, seeds, avocado, and coconut. It is recommended that fats do not exceed 10% of daily dietary intake, and incorporating some raw vegetables is also beneficial. Relying solely on smoothies and juices without including leafy greens in the diet can lead to dental issues over time, as seen in some fruit-only eaters.

Dr. Morse has mentioned reading Arnold Ehret's work in the past, and it is curious why he skips the recommended transitional teachings before advocating for an all-fruit/raw diet. The transitional period is essential for preparing the body and should be explained to individuals with individual attention. However, it can be challenging to teach people how to incorporate a proper transition diet because they often prefer simple instructions on what to eat, when to eat, and how long it will take to heal. Learning the importance of transitioning and taking the necessary time to prepare the body can help avoid unforeseen issues. Deficiency and malabsorption are common concerns, but through hydration and a health-promoting diet/lifestyle, the body can absorb nutrients efficiently once it has eliminated waste and cleaned itself out. Patience and time are key in the healing process.

Transitioning to a raw food diet can indeed be challenging, especially for individuals with a history of consuming disease-forming foods like meat, cheese, milk, and eggs. Cravings for heavier, complex foods can be overwhelming, partly due to the presence of harmful waste residues in the body. In such cases, it may be beneficial to include heavier plant foods like cooked vegetables combined with greens in the diet for a period to help buffer the effects of the cleansing process as the body eliminates pharmaceutical waste.

 As the body becomes cleaner, cravings typically decrease, making it easier to transition to a 100% raw food diet for health and longevity. It is important to note that an all-fruit diet alone may not meet all our dietary needs, as a balance of fruits and leafy greens is essential. Deficiency and malabsorption can be addressed through proper hydration, returning to a health-promoting diet and lifestyle, and allowing the body time to clean out waste and improve nutrient absorption.

While Dr. Robert Morse assists terminally ill patients and cancer patients who may not have much time to gradually transition, it would be beneficial if he recognized the potential harm of herbal substances to varying degrees. Herbal tinctures, especially when processed, can burden and stimulate the body, which is not ideal for overall health. Instead of combining multiple herbs into alcohol tinctures, a more sensible approach would be to use whole, singular herbs if one believed they were health-promoting.

Even if I were to believe today that herbs have health-promoting properties, I would not consider it beneficial to combine multiple herbs into an alcohol tincture for daily consumption. Instead, it would make more sense to teach individuals to use whole, singular herbs if they were deemed helpful. Dr. Morse likely believes that his herbal formulas assist in detoxification and healing, which is why he created his own line of herbal products. However, based on my experience in his online groups, it seems that many individuals approach his protocols as a short-term fix rather than adopting them as a long-term, lifestyle-based approach to health and healing.

It appears that Dr. Morse's protocols have attracted individuals who view health and healing as a short-term fix, rather than adopting a long-term, lifestyle approach. Many people using his protocols have no intention of maintaining the diet that helped them heal or improve their health conditions. This may be due, in part, to Dr. Morse not teaching people how to build healthier long-term dietary and lifestyle habits to prevent future health issues. It is essential to view health and healing as a holistic, long-term approach rather than a fragmented, temporary solution.

When I started working alongside others in our monthly Terrain Model Diet Support Group, I was still including steamed vegetables in my otherwise raw food diet. However, as I began teaching the importance of a fully raw diet for healing and health, I felt a responsibility to lead by example and transition to a 100% raw diet myself. In the previous years I had gone through several periods of 100% raw foods. But It felt wrong to instruct others to do what I was not doing consistently. I had always known that I would eventually take the final step toward being 100% raw, but I was taking my time with the transition. It was the support and influence of the group that motivated me to eliminate the last bit of non-ideal foods from my diet, particularly the lightly steamed vegetables in my evening meal. To my surprise, the difference in my health after eliminating the last bit of cooked food from my diet was remarkable. I had not realized that even a small amount of cooked vegetables could still burden my body. The shift from 80% raw to 100% raw was like night and day, and I have no desire to go back to consuming cooked vegetables because I feel significantly better on a raw diet. Although I may have the occasional small portion of cooked vegetables, it is now a rarity in my eating habits.

Throughout my journey in the health community, I have come to realize the potential for unintentional misinformation, especially when it comes to the concept of detoxification. Detoxification is not something we actively do to our bodies; it is a natural process that our bodies carry out on their own. Focusing solely on detoxification can create a misconception that we have control over the body's healing process and the ability to dictate when and how it cleanses itself.

I have learned that building long-lasting healthy dietary and lifestyle habits is crucial. By doing so, we can support our body's natural healing processes, and the need to overly focus on detoxification diminishes. Healing takes time and cannot be predicted or rushed. This understanding is why many individuals view dietary recommendations for healing and cleansing, such as those promoted by Dr. Morse, as short-term interventions rather than long-term lifestyle choices.

Unfortunately, we have been deprived of valuable information on how to properly care for and nourish our bodies from childhood. However, those who truly understand health recognize that there is no quick-fix diet for healing. Instead, adopting healthier dietary habits and routines over time is essential for sustained health and well-being. Our bodies are designed for specific foods, much like a cow is designed to eat grass.

It may sound surprising, but I have come to question the use of herbs for human health. This realization has led me to explore the principles of Natural Hygiene, which I plan to explain further in a dedicated chapter. Initially, when someone challenged the benefits of herbs in one of my posts, I dismissed their comment without seeking further clarification. It took time for me to acknowledge that I had devoted years of my life to studying incorrect information through herbal and horticulture studies.

To deepen my understanding, I enrolled in Dr. Morse's "Detoxification Specialist" Certificate Program online. Although the course was more of a review for me, it provided a comprehensive understanding of Dr. Morse's teachings. Armed with my certificate, I began working with individuals seeking healing through Dr. Morse's protocols. However, after a couple of years, I noticed that many people were not experiencing the desired results with the herbs. Some even reported feeling worse. Intrigued, I instinctively suggested eliminating the herbs for a few weeks, and the individuals reported feeling better.

Driven by curiosity, I delved into extensive reading on health and healing. I explored the works of authors such as Herbert Shelton, TC Fry, Dr. Doug Graham, R.T. Trall, and others. The writings of Arnold Ehret particularly captivated me, drawing me to older literature from the early 18th and 19th centuries.

My journey of assisting people in reclaiming their health began organically, without me ever envisioning myself as a health coach. Initially, I offered support and guidance on a donation basis. As time passed, I recognized the value of my time and expertise, and I began charging for consultations. To this day, what I find most fulfilling is one-on-one consultations, where I can discuss individuals' unique health goals and concerns. Through these personalized conversations, we work together to determine the best approach for transitioning to a natural diet and lifestyle.

As I continue to learn and grow, my goal is to empower individuals to take control of their health, build lasting habits, and foster a deep understanding of the body's innate healing abilities.

According to Natural Hygiene teachings, herbs, along with spices, salts, vitamins, supplements, powders, and isolates, do not heal the body as commonly believed. Rather, herbs are inert substances, essentially poisons due to their bitter or unfavorable taste, which burden the body and drain our life force energy upon ingestion. It is the body that acts on the herbs, rather than the other way around, and herbs are categorized based on perceived effects on the body, such as diuretics, laxatives, or sedatives, contrary to popular belief.

Grasping this new information on herbs and their effects (or lack thereof) on the body was not easy, given my prior immersion in herbal studies. However, as I delved further into uncovering lies and seeking truth in various areas, I found that often the truth lies in the opposite of what is commonly taught. The simplicity and logic behind Natural Hygiene's perspective resonated with me. Nature wouldn't complicate our lives by requiring us to spend a lifetime deciphering which herbs can help with our self-created health issues.

Additionally, my own observations and experiences working with individuals further reinforced this perspective. I had minimal personal reliance on herbal support throughout my own healing journey, relying primarily on dietary and lifestyle changes. Avoiding herbs not only saved me time and money but also protected my health from potential downgrade. Living in a rural area, I had access to high-quality herbs growing abundantly around me, but I felt instinctively that my dietary and lifestyle changes were sufficient.

Ultimately, everyone must research, think, and decide for themselves. This topic is highly controversial, particularly considering the significant emphasis Dr. Morse places on herbal formulas as support during detoxification. In my coaching experiences, I encountered cases where herbal formulas did not yield the desired results, and individuals themselves expressed skepticism about their effectiveness. Some reported improvements in their health after temporarily discontinuing herbal use.

While I acknowledge that my experience and observations do not constitute a formal case study or scientific research, I share these insights based on my personal journey. Many years ago, I briefly tried Dr. Morse's herbal tinctures while following a raw fruit diet, but my intuition led me to abandon their use. Instead, if I were to use herbs, I preferred single herbs that I could grow or forage myself, as it seemed like a healthier option. Dr. Morse's herbal tinctures contain a combination of at least nine different herbs, and I believe that such complex mixtures, regardless of their perceived harmlessness, carry risks. The interactions between specific herbs and their concentration within the body remain difficult to ascertain.

I understand that some long-time followers of Dr. Morse may perceive my previous comments as a personal attack on him. I want to assure everyone that it is not my intention. Dr. Morse is a well-intentioned individual who has helped many people on their healing journeys. However, I believe that he may only have a partial understanding of the truth.

In my exploration of health and healing, I came across new information that challenged my beliefs about the effectiveness of herbal potions. This was a significant blow to me personally, as I had invested years studying and advocating herbal medicine. The realization that herbs may not be as beneficial as I once thought was difficult to accept. Nevertheless, I still appreciate the beauty and properties of herbs; I just no longer feel the need to incorporate them into my own healing practices.

In my upcoming chapter "Natural Hygiene", I will delve deeper into the topic of herbs and present a more comprehensive exploration of their effects and the principles that guide my perspective. It is important to continue the discussion on this controversial topic, as it has significant implications for our understanding of health and healing.

One aspect of Dr. Morse's teachings that I highly value is his ability to simplify complex concepts and make them accessible to a wide audience. His explanations of the lymphatic system and the body's detoxification processes during illness are clear and easy to understand. He encourages individuals to consider the true causes of disease, which are often related to our dietary and lifestyle choices rather than external factors like germs.

Dr. Morse provides compelling evidence that our anatomy and physiology are designed for a frugivorous diet, drawing comparisons between our teeth and those of true carnivores. This resonates with me because the truth is often simple and easy to understand. Through my own healing journey and witnessing others heal through a return to our species-appropriate diet and lifestyle changes, I have seen the power of adopting a natural approach to health.

Dr. Morse has built a significant following over the years and recently established a dedicated school to spread his teachings. People from around the world attend his classes, both online and in person, and his methods are gaining popularity. It is evident from the thriving nature of his business that he has positively impacted the lives of countless individuals.

In my personal experience with Dr. Morse's information, I have had nothing but positive results. However, I attribute this in part to already having a foundation in a transitional diet, which is crucial to avoid falling back into old dietary habits once the body begins eliminating waste and experiencing symptom relief.

Dr. Morse appears to be a genuine and kind-hearted individual, and his ability to trigger individuals' ability, desire, and motivation to heal themselves is what makes him a great healer in my eyes. Many of those who find success in healing themselves are individuals who have exhausted all mainstream options and are willing to explore more fundamental and simplistic approaches to health. They realize that sometimes doing things less intelligently is the key, even though it may seem counterintuitive.

Ultimately, we must continue to evolve and refine our understanding of health and healing as new information presents itself. It is essential to critically examine and question our beliefs, even those we hold dear, to continually improve and help others on their healing journeys.

Chapter 6
Dr. John McDougall: A Pioneer in Healing Through Starch-Based Nutrition

Dr. John McDougall, an esteemed American physician, renowned author, and captivating speaker, has dedicated his life to promoting the transformative power of a whole-food, starch-based diet for preventing, reversing, and healing chronic diseases. His groundbreaking work has impacted countless individuals worldwide, helping them improve their health, shed excess weight, and overcome serious health issues such as heart disease, diabetes, obesity, arthritis, and more.

Born on May 17, 1947, Dr. McDougall's journey into the world of medicine took a remarkable turn due to a life-altering event in his early years. At just 18 years old, he experienced a massive stroke that left him temporarily paralyzed on his left side for two weeks. This profound incident, though challenging, served as the catalyst that drove him towards a career in medicine. He realized that he wanted to be a healer, someone who could make a meaningful difference in the lives of others.

Dr. McDougall's medical education began in 1965, and he embarked on a transformative path of discovery and learning. During his internship at Queens Medical Centre in Honolulu on Oahu, he assumed a pivotal role as one of four medical doctors responsible for the health and well-being of 5000 people, including the laborers and their families at the Hamakua sugar plantation.

Through his diverse medical duties, ranging from delivering babies to signing death certificates, Dr. McDougall observed that traditional medical approaches often fell short in treating chronic health issues. Conventional pills and prescriptions appeared ineffective, and he became increasingly curious about the root causes of these widespread ailments plaguing the Western World.

It was during his tenure at the Hamakua sugar plantation, between 1973 and 1976, that Dr. McDougall made a groundbreaking discovery. He noticed a striking correlation between diet and disease among his elderly patients who had immigrated to Hawaii from countries like China, Japan, Philippines, and Korea. In their home countries, rice (starch) was a staple in their diets, and they remained healthy and vibrant well into their 90s, free from common Western diseases.

However, subsequent generations who adopted Westernized diets witnessed a significant decline in their health. Their children and grandchildren suffered from obesity and a range of chronic diseases prevalent in the Western World. Dr. McDougall's keen observations led him to the conclusion that a diet primarily based on starch and vegetable foods could be the key to promoting optimal health and preventing chronic ailments.

Dr. McDougall's passion for educating others about the profound diet-disease connection led him to write several national best-selling books. Among his most acclaimed works is "The Starch Solution," a book that has become a cornerstone for individuals seeking to improve their health through a starch-based, low-fat, vegan diet.

Throughout his illustrious career spanning over four decades, Dr. John McDougall has been a staunch advocate for his dietary philosophy, known as the "McDougall Plan." The plan has withstood the test of time and became a New York Times bestseller, further solidifying his influence on health-conscious individuals worldwide.

Beyond his literary contributions, Dr. McDougall has appeared in the influential documentary "Forks Over Knives," which has brought his revolutionary ideas to a broader audience. Additionally, he teamed up with his wife, Mary, to establish "Dr. McDougall's Right Foods Grocery Product Line," offering healthy and convenient food options aligned with his dietary principles.

Dr. McDougall's biography is a testament to his unwavering dedication to improving human health through the power of a starch-based diet. His journey from a life-changing stroke to becoming a leading figure in the field of plant-based nutrition serves as an inspiring narrative of resilience, passion, and the pursuit of a healthier world.

For a more comprehensive account of Dr. John McDougall's life, background, and remarkable achievements, one can explore his website at www.DrMcDougall.com, where his fascinating story continues to inspire countless individuals to embrace the transformative potential of plant-based nutrition.

The Starch Solution Diet

Dr. John McDougall's dietary recommendations are centered around a whole-food, plant-based diet that he calls the "Starch Solution." He believes that human beings are naturally "Starchitarians," and that a diet predominantly based on starches is optimal for our health and well-being. His dietary guidelines emphasize high-fiber, low-fat, minimally processed, and vegan foods, while avoiding animal products, processed oils, and fats of all kinds.

The core of Dr. McDougall's diet consists of approximately 90% starch-based foods, such as potatoes, rice (brown, white, or wild), corn, whole grains, pasta, tortillas, and legumes. Dr. McDougall believes that these starches serve as the foundation for providing essential nutrients, sustained energy, and promoting satiety.

The remaining 10% of the diet comprises what he calls "supplementary" foods, including whole fruits, vegetables, and leafy greens. These foods offer additional vitamins, minerals, and phytonutrients to complement the starch-based diet.

Dr. McDougall is a vocal advocate for addressing what he refers to as "food poisoning" on a global scale. He believes that many preventable diseases stem from poor dietary choices, with people unwittingly causing harm to their health while attributing their sickness to external factors like germs. In his view, the key to better health lies in adopting a plant-based diet that avoids harmful elements present in animal products, processed foods, and unhealthy fats.

The Starch Solution Diet is designed to be accessible and easy to incorporate into modern lifestyles. Starch-based foods are readily available in grocery stores and restaurants, making it convenient for people to follow the diet. Dr. McDougall encourages the use of condiments to enhance the flavors of starch foods, as he believes that making the diet enjoyable and palatable increases adherence. These condiments include items like vinegars, salt, organic brown sugar, agave, maple syrup, nutritional yeast, ketchup, mustard, and various herbs and spices.

In line with his whole-food philosophy, Dr. McDougall does not generally recommend the use of dietary supplements. However, he acknowledges the importance of vitamin B12, which is primarily found in animal-based foods. As a precaution, he suggests taking a B12 supplement to ensure sufficient intake, even though he believes most people can obtain this "nutrient" through a healthy plant based diet.

Overall, Dr. John McDougall's dietary recommendations advocate for a sustainable, health-promoting lifestyle that revolves around a starch-based, plant-focused diet, contributing to better overall health and well-being.

As I ventured deeper into the realms of dietary exploration, I found myself drawn to the idea of incorporating whole food plant starches into my meals for experimentation purposes. I decided to give the Starch Solution Diet (SSD) a trial. Little did I realize that this dietary experiment would lead me to question the extent of starch's role in my long-term health and longevity.

Reasons I Decided to Try Dr. John McDougall's Starch Solution Diet:

Approximately 7-8 years into my journey of following a high raw, mucusless diet, complemented by occasional fasting and 100% raw phases, I found myself contemplating a dietary experiment— the "Starch Solution Diet" by Dr. John McDougall. After listening to countless Dr. John McDougall lectures and reading his works, curiosity led me to embark on a 100-day trial of this diet, a period of self-experimentation to explore its potential benefits and effects on my well-being. Several reasons influenced my decision to make this dietary change:

1. Exploration and Learning: As someone deeply interested in health and nutrition, I saw this as an opportunity to expand my knowledge and understanding of different dietary approaches. I was open to exploring new perspectives and wanted to experience firsthand the touted benefits of the Starch Solution Diet.

2. Filling Nutritional Gaps: While my previous diet had served me well for many years, I wondered if incorporating more starches into my meals would provide additional satiety and fill any potential nutritional gaps in my existing diet.

3. Community Influence: The growing popularity of the Starch Solution Diet among health enthusiasts and its endorsements from various advocates prompted my curiosity. I wanted to understand why so many people found success and improvement in their health on this plan.

4. A Transition Diet: I considered the Starch Solution Diet as a potential transition away from certain processed foods and animal products. I believed it could be a gentler approach for individuals under my guidance who were seeking to adopt a plant-based diet but not ready to embrace a fully raw or extreme regimen.

5. Addressing Cravings: While I thoroughly enjoyed my high raw, healthy vegan diet, I occasionally experienced cravings for heartier and more substantial meals. I hoped that incorporating starches might help satisfy these cravings while maintaining a 100% plant-based approach.

6. Balancing Health and Taste: I wondered if striking a balance between optimal health and culinary pleasure could be achieved through the Starch Solution Diet. The prospect of indulging in comforting starch-based dishes while adhering to plant-based principles was enticing.

7. Alignment with Previous Studies: Dr. McDougall's information on coffee, salt, oil, sugar, vitamins/supplements, etc. matched what I had already studied and learned. His insights resonated with my existing knowledge.

8. Curiosity about Starches: Having avoided starch for eight years due to concerns from Arnold Ehret, Natural Hygiene, Dr. Robert Morse, and others, I wanted to test if the natural breakdown of starch into simple sugars was as burdensome on overall health as claimed.

9. Seeking Direct Experience: Embracing the Starch Solution Diet allowed me to personally experience its effects and uncover the truth about starches and their impact on human health.

With these reasons in mind, I embarked on my 100-day trial with an open mind and a desire to explore the potential benefits and drawbacks of the Starch Solution Diet. Little did I know that this experiment would lead me to discover profound insights about my body, health, and solidify in my mind what the optimal diet for health truly was.

For the past eight years, my diet has revolved around fruits, greens, and vegetables, with minimal plant fats like avocado or coconut. While I occasionally indulged in less-than-ideal vegan options, my commitment to this wholesome diet remained steadfast. Transitioning to the Starch Solution Diet meant eliminating plant fats entirely, including avocado, tahini, and coconut, while incorporating whole starch foods—an entirely new food group for me. As I embarked on this path, I found myself resisting the permitted condiments, feeling that it would be a step backward from the progress I had made in the past.

Dr. McDougall's assertion that fats are non-beneficial foods resonated with me, and I felt a positive shift in my digestion and overall well-being. Having experimented with periods of zero fat consumption during my years of practicing the Mucusless Diet Healing System, I recognized the benefits of avoiding fats in the diet as they are considered "mucus forming foods" which is easily felt when overdoing them. Adjusting to the addition of starches to my existing fruits, greens, and vegetables was a significant shift. I must admit that eliminating plant fats from my meals was a challenge, as they had been the base of my salad dressings for quite some time. However, I heeded the call to follow Dr. McDougall's dietary recommendations and persevered.

My daily routine on the Starch Solution Diet included a freshly made fruit juice, usually orange, to kickstart my eating window around noon. Lunchtime brought a large salad topped with steamed vegetables and a starch item such as rice, potatoes, a sprouted whole wheat wrap, or corn tortillas, representing approximately one-third of my meal. Dr. McDougall's recommendation of making starch 90% of the plate seemed excessive to me, and I adjusted the ratio to suit my preferences.

After 75 days on the Starch Solution Diet, I observed some intriguing effects. Starch proved to be satiating, leaving me satisfied after a meal without craving additional food. Interestingly, by dinner, I often found myself eating fruit not out of hunger but a genuine love for its health benefits. However, I couldn't help but miss the clarity of mind I had experienced with my previous diet, as starch seemed to cause a slight brain fog.

Throughout this dietary exploration, I remained attuned to my body's needs and sought to mitigate any adverse effects. Drinking adequate water was crucial, as I realized starch could lead to constipation and dehydration without proper hydration. Additionally, while I initially hoped for remarkable health improvements as Dr. McDougall's claims suggested, my experience didn't align with his "Starchitarian" philosophy. I couldn't ignore the teachings of Dr. Robert Morse, Natural Hygiene, and Professor Arnold Ehret, who championed a "fruitarian" approach.

The transition to the Starch Solution Diet from my longstanding mucusless diet didn't seem challenging at first, as I was merely adding whole starches to my existing regimen of fruits, greens, and vegetables. However, as the days progressed, I started noticing unsettling changes in my body. Bloating and constipation, which had been rare on my previous diet, became regular occurrences. My mood shifted, and I experienced frequent headaches. After experiencing a week-long headache that left me feeling overwhelmed and depleted it was time for another change. I couldn't deny that these symptoms that I was experiencing aligned with the introduction of starches to my diet.

What began as a hopeful experiment turned into a profound revelation about the impact of starches on my body and well-being. Throughout the experiment, I embraced the SSD's emphasis on plain whole foods, finding contentment in the simplicity of unadorned flavors. Unlike many proponents of the diet who rely on condiments to stay engaged, I preferred the natural taste of my meals and avoided processed additions like sugar, salt, vinegars, and nutritional yeast. My focus was on nourishing my body with pure, unaltered foods.

As I continued, I reminded myself that dietary changes take time to manifest in health, but my intuition nagged at me. I had experienced positive healing outcomes from my previous diet, and this deviation seemed to lead me in the opposite direction. The 75-day mark approached, and my body cried out for a change. It craved the digestive rest and the abundance of water-rich raw foods it had once thrived on.

While I had hoped that rice, pasta, beans, and breads would prove healthy options, my personal experience contradicted this. I longed for a greater improvement in my well-being, but it never came. Starches left me feeling bloated, constipated, and moody, impacting my skin and even my teeth. The dental plaque I had managed to eliminate with my previous dietary habits/routines returned, and my teeth lost their previous luster.

A profound moment came when my old earlobe piercing holes became red, swollen, and sore, a familiar sign of inflammation that I hadn't experienced in years. My body was clearly telling me that the Starch Solution Diet wasn't serving its needs.

As I sit here, reflecting on my 75-day experience with Dr. John McDougall's Starch Solution Diet, I can't help but acknowledge the twists and turns this journey has taken. Initially aiming for a full 100-day trial, I find myself unable to proceed further. This chapter of my health exploration has been filled with eye-opening revelations and challenges that have left me questioning my long-held dietary beliefs.

Though I wished starches were a healthy addition to my diet, I couldn't ignore my body's signals. As I move forward, I plan to resume my preferred fruit and greens high raw diet, which has supported my health for years. Starches, it seems, are not the right fit for my body, and I am grateful for this complete awareness.

I want to emphasize that my experience might not be representative of everyone's reaction to the Starch Solution Diet. Each body is unique, and it really depends on where we are starting from and our level of health. I genuinely believe in giving any diet a fair trial, and my 75-day journey on the SSD was an honest attempt to explore its potential. Ultimately, my body's response guided me back to my preferred path. While some may find the SSD beneficial coming from a previous diet of processed foods and animal products, I discovered that it wasn't suitable for me. I will remain open to dietary exploration, however, I'm content to return 100% to the diet that brought me optimal health and well-being.

In the initial stages of my SSD journey, I discovered that starch foods could serve as a valuable transition group for those seeking to bid farewell to harmful foods such as meat, dairy, and eggs. They provided a sense of satiation and helped assuage those inevitable cravings. However, I quickly realized that relying on starch as the foundation of my diet, especially at the overwhelming 90% recommended by Dr. McDougall was not the path I wished to follow.

Instead, I began viewing starches as occasional and supplementary additions to a health promoting diet. Focusing on health-promoting raw fruits, greens, and vegetables is my top priority. My recommendation for anyone including starches in their diet is to eat them in moderation, always paired with a leafy green salad for improved digestion.

For individuals transitioning from a diet laden with standard foods like animal products and processed items, the SSD can prove beneficial. By eliminating complex and other non-health-promoting foods, the body often experiences an overall improvement in well-being, leading many to attribute these positive changes solely to starches.

Arnold Ehret's cautionary remarks about starches possessing "sticky gluey properties" that hindered proper elimination began resonating deeply with me again because I experienced the effects firsthand. Although I agreed with Ehret's statements more than ever, I couldn't help but acknowledge the initial surprise I experienced at how digestible these starch foods seemed in the beginning of my experiment. This, I concluded, was largely attributed to pairing them with a salad for better digestion.

UPDATE:

After the 75-day ordeal with the Starch Solution Diet, I found myself seeking solace in the simplicity of raw fruits and greens. It seemed my body had much to clear and cleanse after the heavy burden of daily starch consumption. During these past two weeks, my appetite naturally diminished as my body focused on eliminating internal waste accumulated during the SSD experiment.

My current routine revolves around the nourishing power of water fasting until noon, followed by a revitalizing freshly squeezed orange juice. An hour later, I indulged in my signature raw apple sauce—a delightful blend of dates and apples topped with raisins or fresh fruit. For dinner, a generous serving of fresh salad with homemade dressing leaves me satiated and content.

The effects of this raw fruit and greens regimen were evident almost immediately. My health had begun to improve, and I felt a renewed sense of well-being. My skin, once dry and lackluster during my 75-day SSD trial, started to regain its vitality. The inflammation and redness in my piercing holes that lingered since the SSD days were now nearly gone. Even my teeth were gradually regaining their natural whiteness, and the plaque that built during my SSD trial was fading away.

Sleep, one of the pillars of good health, had once again become a peaceful sanctuary for me. Restful nights and improved moods were welcome companions, replacing the headaches and negative thoughts that plagued my days after the initial "honeymoon period" on the Starch Solution Diet.

Reflecting on my experience, I couldn't help but appreciate the significance of listening to my body's signals. It craved less food after eliminating starches, signaling the need to allow it time and space to heal from the inflammation caused by the daily consumption of starchy foods. Through patience and attentive care, I have given my body the chance to restore its balance.

Months after my SSD experiment, I can confidently say that my health has returned to its former state, and I've put the painful headaches and starch-induced discomfort behind me. The experiment was worthwhile in affirming my belief that starch foods can be dehydrating and constipating for the human body.

To anyone considering the Starch Solution Diet, I would recommend it as a temporary transition away from other harmful foods. It can be a useful steppingstone towards a healthier path, especially for those seeking a gentler approach to change. However, in my quest for optimal health and disease-free living, I've come to realize that our species-appropriate diet consists of raw fruits, non-starchy vegetables, leafy greens, and a small amount of plant-based fats from nuts, seeds, and avocado.

As Arnold Ehret wisely put it, "The truth is simple," and indeed, the natural human diet is no exception. Through this journey, I've learned to trust my body's wisdom and to embrace simplicity as the foundation of true well-being.

Chapter 7
Natural Hygiene - Embracing Healthful Living

In the realm of health and wellness, one approach stands apart as a timeless and scientifically grounded system - Natural Hygiene. Rooted in centuries of scientific analysis and observation, this branch of biology revolves around the preservation and restoration of health. In today's world, where unhealthy lifestyles and dietary practices abound, Natural Hygiene offers a guiding light back to the fundamentals of well-being.

The term "Hygiene" finds its origins in *"Hygiea,"* the Greek Goddess of Health, and it represents the conditions and practices that foster well-being. At its core, Natural Hygiene recognizes the human body's remarkable capacity for self-healing and maintenance of health when its basic needs are met. The essence of genuine health lies in living healthfully, and Natural Hygiene endeavors to help us relearn what it means to lead a wholesome life.

One crucial principle of Natural Hygiene is the understanding that there are no magical "cures" for ailments. Instead, the focus is on restoring health by relinquishing enervating habits. By identifying these habits and learning to let go of them, one can set themselves on a path to rejuvenation and lasting vitality. This lifestyle is not merely a method of treatment but a profound way of nourishing the body and making wise choices.

The roots of Natural Hygiene can be traced back to the early 1830s when forward-thinking medical doctors began to question and abandon the traditional drugging and medical practices of their time. The term *"Hygiene"* or *"Orothopathy"* emerged from this growing movement as these pioneers sought a more natural and holistic approach to health and well-being.

In its essence, Natural Hygiene teaches that optimal health cannot be achieved through dietary changes alone. Instead, it involves a harmonious integration of various pillars of health that collectively influence our well-being. From proper nutrition to exercise, sleep, stress management, and more - each aspect plays a vital role in our overall health. Every aspect plays a crucial role in achieving and maintaining optimal health, as Natural Hygiene teaches.

Our current state of health reflects the choices we make daily, as they accumulate over time to shape our well-being. To truly achieve and maintain optimal health, Natural Hygiene encourages us to align ourselves with the wisdom of Natural Law. It calls for a return to our species-appropriate foods in their raw state, acknowledging that our bodies are designed to thrive on nourishment that aligns with our true requirements. By delving into the principles of Natural Hygiene, we can discover the secrets of building and maintaining health. This approach advocates not just a fleeting fix but a lifelong journey of healthful living. As we learn to honor the intrinsic needs of the human organism, we unlock the potential for greater vitality, youthfulness, longevity, and an improved quality of life.

Studying the principles of Natural Hygiene enables us to build a strong foundation of health and learn how to sustain it. By living in accordance with the wisdom of Natural Law, we can unlock the secrets to longevity, vitality, and true well-being. The journey toward optimal health beckons, and it starts with the embrace of Natural Hygiene—a time-honored approach to healthy living.

In the pursuit of optimal health and vitality, Natural Hygiene emerges as a profound revelation—one that delves into the core principles of human well-being. At its essence lies the understanding that humans are inherently classified as "Frugivores." Returning to our species-appropriate foods, in their raw and unadulterated form, combined with a health-promoting lifestyle, is the key to restoring the body's natural balance and vibrant health. The body, in its innate wisdom, always strives for balance and well-being, but it is our enervating habits and choices that hinder its path towards a healthy state.

Natural Hygiene firmly asserts that there are no quick fixes or magic remedies to address the root cause of our ailments. No substance, herb, vitamin, supplement, powder, isolate, pharmaceutical, or pill can replace the body's own healing capabilities. Only when we provide the correct conditions and diet can the body truly heal itself.

At the heart of Natural Hygiene lies the fundamental belief that every living creature, including humankind, is naturally designed for a specific set of foods. These foods serve as the anatomical foundation for thriving health and a life free from disease.

The human body is intrinsically designed to run on carbohydrates, particularly simple sugars, contrary to prevailing mainstream beliefs. Embracing our classification as "Frugivores," our natural diet predominantly consists of fruits, leafy-tender greens, non-starchy vegetables, and minimal nuts/seeds or plant fats. This diet fulfills all our dietary needs without burdening the body's digestive system with excessive work.

Within the wisdom of Natural Hygiene, disease issues and symptoms are not shrouded in mystery. Through diligent study and comprehension of its teachings and principles, one can understand that diseases develop and are built through our daily dietary and lifestyle choices—not contracted as suggested by the "Germ Theory" promoted in mainstream medical science. The roots of Natural Hygiene reach far beyond the early 1850s, representing a wealth of ancient knowledge that is not new but has been overshadowed by contemporary beliefs.

Central to Natural Hygiene's understanding is the "Terrain Model," which places emphasis on the connection between diet and disease, highlighting cause and effect. This model resonates more authentically than the widely accepted "Germ Theory," which tends to attribute sickness to external sources, absolving individuals of personal responsibility and accountability for their health.

The allure of the germ theory narrative is rooted in the perception that germs, as an outside force, bear the blame for illness, providing a comforting detachment from personal habits and routines. However, a closer examination of this perspective reveals its limitations. If germ theory were entirely accurate, humanity would be perpetually plagued by illness, with no exception for even the healthiest individuals.

This leads us to a critical revelation—our current state of health is intrinsically linked to the state of our inner terrain and how the body responds to exposure to toxins. Armed with this knowledge, Natural Hygiene encourages us to reclaim ownership of our well-being, empowering us to make conscious choices and adopt a lifestyle that fosters optimal health from within.

In the world of Natural Hygiene, a fundamental debate rages between the Germ Theory and the Terrain Model. The Germ Theory model has not only served as the basis for the pharmaceutical industry but also provided a convenient excuse for the creation and use of pharmaceutical drugs. However, many have come to question the efficacy of pharmaceuticals, as they seem to merely suppress symptoms, driving them deeper within the body and potentially leading to chronic and degenerative conditions over time.

The prevailing belief among most people today is that germs are the primary cause of illness or disease. This perception conveniently absolves individuals of accountability for their health, attributing the blame to an external source. However, within the principles of Natural Hygiene, this belief is challenged, as it highlights the crucial role of individual habits and choices in determining health outcomes.

A central focus of Natural Hygiene is our diet—a true Natural Diet that aligns with the health requirements of our species. Deviating from our species appropriate diet weakens the body and renders it susceptible to toxicity issues and symptomatic states. Over time, such deviations may culminate in chronic and degenerative conditions. What we consume daily has a profound impact on our overall health; hence, we must take responsibility for the choices we make, as they directly contribute to creating our own diseases.

Within the Facebook group "Terrain Model Refutes Germ Theory," an ever-growing community of over 33K members passionately explores the wisdom of Natural Hygiene and the Terrain Model. This group, meticulously moderated by dedicated individuals, offers an incredible library filled with invaluable resources on the subject. The thirst for this knowledge is evident, as people seek to understand the profound implications of Natural Hygiene on their well-being.

As part of this mission, I collaborate with Lauren Whiteman and

Nat Farris to support and guide individuals through our paid subscription group, "The Terrain Model Diet Support Group." For a nominal fee of $20, members gain access to ongoing teachings and guidance throughout the month, empowering them to build healthier, sustainable, long-term habits. The satisfaction derived from helping others achieve optimal health and knowledge is immeasurable, as we believe that well-being should be every individual's birthright.

The debate between the Germ Theory and the Terrain Model resonates at the core of Natural Hygiene. By questioning prevailing beliefs and embracing the principles of Natural Hygiene, we empower ourselves to take charge of our health and well-being. The profound wisdom of the Terrain Model inspires us to delve deeper into the science of life and natural healing. Together, as a community, we unravel the truth and embark on a journey towards a healthier, more fulfilled life.

Within the thriving Facebook group titled "Terrain Model Refutes Germ Theory," a team of dedicated moderators, including myself, work tirelessly to curate an exceptional library filled with invaluable resources on Natural Hygiene and the Terrain Model. This group has witnessed remarkable growth, attracting over 33K members who thirst for knowledge and seek to understand the profound implications of the Terrain Model.

As a moderator, I contribute to the group by providing valuable insights, answering questions, and fostering discussions among members. Despite our best efforts, the sheer activity and engagement within the group can be overwhelming, a testament to the immense interest in this life-transforming knowledge.

For me, dedicating time and energy to these groups is an honor and a deeply rewarding experience. There is nothing more fulfilling than helping others achieve the health and knowledge that rightfully belongs to every individual. The thirst for understanding and the desire to reclaim ownership of one's well-being is palpable within the community, motivating us to continue sharing the profound wisdom of Natural Hygiene.

As we unite as a community, we unravel the truths concealed by the prevalent Germ Theory narrative. Our mission is to empower individuals to break free from limiting beliefs and embrace the

Terrain Model to rediscover their body's innate healing abilities. By cultivating healthier lifestyles and fostering a deep connection with nature, we forge a path towards optimal health and fulfillment.

The following was a collaborative effort written by friends that moderate the Facebook group, "Terrain Model Refutes Germ Theory":

"The Germ Theory of disease creation claims that microorganisms invade the body and that this is what causes disease. Despite the passage of more than 150 years, it has still not been scientifically verified. When subjected to credible third-party testing, the evidence supporting the Germ Theory fails to prove that any germ is the direct cause of any disease.

The Terrain Model is a disease model which states that the state of the Terrain (the internal condition of the body) is the cause of dis-ease within the body. The Terrain Model disproves Germ Theory which states that external invading "germs" are the cause of disease. The Terrain Model began out of the Terrain Theory of Antoine Bechamp and his contemporaries, with the discovery of Pleomorphism and the idea that "the germ is nothing, the terrain is everything".

The Terrain Theory of Disease Creation was expanded and refined over the following 150+ years, through the work of Natural Hygienists and the Study of Life Science. Through extensive clinical research, these scientists observed a correlation between disease creation and the number of toxins a person was exposed to, through diet and environmental factors. These disease conditions were then observed to reverse themselves when the diet and lifestyle conditions were corrected by a return to the natural, fruit-centered diet.

The Natural Hygienists also observed that there are two forms of disease symptoms, Constructive Symptoms and Malfunction Symptoms. Constructive symptoms are symptoms like "colds" and "flus", where the body is expelling toxins and waste. Malfunction symptoms are when the body has moved into a Chronic state where the wastes (toxemia) are affecting the function of an organ or gland.

The Hygienists observed that when a body was returned to the natural fruit-centered diet, the malfunction symptoms would move into the Constructive Symptoms through the healing phase and then if the person remained on the fruit-based diet, the constructive symptoms would also be eliminated and would not return as long as Terrain remained clean. Thus proving "Le microbe n'est rien, le terrain est tout." (The microbe is nothing, the terrain is everything) The last words of Louis Pasteur, the father of the Germ Theory.

The Science of Natural Hygiene/Terrain Model has been drowned out by a profit-centered disease industry, creating confusion in marketing and leading the average human into thinking that disease is a mystery and unsure what to do to reverse disease. We hope to clear the confusion by providing the solid foundation of evidence which has been compiled by the Natural Hygienists/ Life Scientists/Nutritionists over the last 200+ years." --Written by Lauren Whiteman and Nathaniel Farris.

Starting in November 2022, Lauren Whiteman, Nat Farris, and I joined forces to moderate the Terrain Model Support Group, dedicated to helping people transition to and maintain a healthy diet and lifestyle based on Natural Hygienic principles. This inclusive group welcomes various plant-based disciplines and provides daily information, inspirational posts, a raw recipe guide, grocery lists, and unlimited Q&A support. We are proud to witness the group grow and thrive as more individuals discover the proper way to care for themselves. If you're interested in joining our ongoing monthly support group, visit therawkey.com or contact me directly at maria@applediaries.com, or through Facebook or Instagram.

 We believe it's unnecessary to spend a lifetime searching for the right dietary information, especially when health concerns are at stake. Many people end up looking in the wrong places, hoping to find healing solutions. Some discover the "cold hard truth" about proper nutrition but find it daunting to embrace a new lifestyle. However, those who embrace Natural Hygienic principles and persist through challenging times are greatly rewarded with vibrant health and abundance. It takes effort, but the rewards are worth it in the long run.

Over the past years of adopting *The Mucusless Diet Healing System*, my focus initially wasn't solely on Natural Hygienic principles. However, I stumbled upon bits and pieces of this path through writings and quotes from pioneers like Herbert Shelton, TC Fry, and Dr. J.H. Tilden. At first, Natural Hygiene's dietary recommendations seemed extreme and strict, as I hadn't fully understood its principles without reading a comprehensive textbook on the subject.

As I delved deeper and gained a better understanding of Natural Hygiene, I realized there were fundamental differences between its teachings and other health information I had encountered on my 9+ year health journey. While I continue to study and learn, I firmly believe that Natural Hygiene is the ultimate guide for caring for and nourishing ourselves as Nature intended. I feel fortunate that I began my journey with learning *The Mucusless Diet Healing System* because after 8 years incorporating the "Transition Diet" I was able to transition to 100% raw with ease.

Over the course of my almost 10-year health journey, I've diligently studied various authors, healers, and advocates of healthy living to find the correct dietary and lifestyle information for my own healing and to help others. Initially, I was greatly influenced by Arnold Ehret's teachings, considering them the most crucial insights on health. However, my perspective shifted when I delved into the principles of Natural Hygiene. Today, I believe that the knowledge I have acquired from Natural Hygiene and Arnold Ehret holds equal importance when it comes to understanding and achieving genuine health and wellness. Through my exploration of Natural Hygiene, I discovered important topics for healthful living and healing that had been largely overlooked in the books I've read and the health circles I've been part of over the past decade. These teachings have opened new horizons and enriched my understanding of holistic well-being.

Here are four essential topics that I've learned from studying Natural Hygiene, which are often overlooked in other health groups, but have had a significant impact on building and maintaining true health:

1. **Working with the body**: In Natural Hygiene, we prioritize listening to the body and allowing it to rest when needed, especially during times of cleaning and repair. Overexertion is avoided, and we aim to lift the burden from the body

wherever possible, understanding that digestion and healing are complex processes.

2. **Simplicity and proper nutrition**: The Terrain model emphasizes the importance of what we put into our bodies. While many health groups focus on this, it's crucial to recognize that both fruits and leafy greens are essential for optimal health. Fruits and greens complement each other, fulfilling the body's nutritional requirements.

3. **Avoiding poisons**: In the Terrain model, we learn to recognize and avoid substances that burden the body. For example, certain herbs and spices can create a burden on the body, hindering the healing process. Understanding what truly poisons the body allows us to return to simplicity and support our body's natural detoxification abilities.

4. **Hydration:** Natural Hygiene underscores the significance of proper water intake, a topic often overlooked in some health groups, even fruitarian circles. Adequate hydration is crucial for achieving desired health results, as fruits alone may not meet all the body's hydration needs in today's world.

By addressing these topics and embracing the principles of Natural Hygiene, we can elevate our health to higher levels and unlock the power of simplicity in nourishing our bodies for true well-being.

I used to think that fruits alone could meet our hydration needs, but I've come to realize that our species-appropriate diet is a diet of hydration. Unfortunately, most of us were raised on diets full of dehydrating foods. Our bodies require about 80% water content for food to move through the digestive tract without pulling water from our cells. It's astonishing to think how dehydrated we might be on a cellular level.

Apart from fruits, greens, and high-water content vegetables, all other foods dehydrate the body to some extent, leading to a dehydrated lymphatic system. A dehydrated lymphatic system can result in various health issues over time. When we talk about constipation issues, it's not just limited to the colon and GI tract; the entire lymphatic system can become constipated and sluggish due to dehydration from unnatural foods and lifestyle choices.

Dehydration caused by consuming water-deficient foods forces the body to draw hydration from its cells to aid digestion. Understanding the importance of proper water intake was a significant revelation for me. Despite having an aversion to drinking water for years, I now believe that my chronic dehydration issues could have been less severe had I been taught to drink more water. Over time, I've come to realize that those who have the greatest aversion to water often need it the most.

Natural Hygiene teaches us these crucial health aspects, often overlooked in the health community, and I'm grateful to share what I've learned so far. It is recommended that we drink 1-1.5 gallons of water per day on average. I admit it was challenging at first, as I had to use the bathroom frequently, but this eventually passed after a couple of months.

My daily water intake routine has been a game-changer for my health. I start my day by drinking two liters of clean distilled water before my first meal, which consists of fresh fruits like oranges, watermelon, or cantaloupe around noon. If I'm still hungry, I might have another fruit meal an hour later, and I stop eating by 2 pm to give my digestive system a break until dinner at 6 pm. My dinner is a large raw leafy green salad with a homemade dressing. This routine, along with my daily workout, has helped me feel my best.

Drinking adequate water has had a profound impact on my health. I noticed my chronic stagnation lifting throughout my body, and my digestion has improved significantly. While I'm still working towards the recommended 1.5-gallon intake, drinking just under a gallon daily has already shown remarkable results. I experienced a detox phase where my body pushed out toxins through my skin, causing temporary rashes and dryness, but it eventually cleared up, leaving me looking healthier and more vibrant.

Frequent urination, a sign of passing toxins, is an inconvenience but an essential part of the detox process. It took about a month or two for it to settle down. I am immensely grateful for discovering the Natural Hygienic principles, as they have improved my health and allowed me to live free from any health issues. I thank those who came before me for sharing this life-saving information and those who continue to spread it to help others achieve vibrant health.

Of all the books I've read on Natural Hygiene, authors like Herbert Shelton, Dr. J.H. Tilden, and T.C. Fry, the teachings are rational and easy to understand. While they may appear radical to some, it's because we no longer live in accordance with Natural Hygienic principles or Natural Law. Most people today eat anything available, from fast food to processed foods. But the truth is simple: a Hygienic diet consists of whole fruits, vegetables, greens, and minimal nuts/seeds/whole plant fats without cooking or processing. Our diet ideally consists of 50% fruit and 50% greens. Some principles include eating slowly, enjoying food, and eating only when calm and joyful. While the Hygienic diet might seem extreme to meat-eaters, it was the original "Vegan" or "Raw Food Diet." Humans may have turned to eating meat out of desperation for survival, but now we have created traditions and holidays centered around eating animals, despite the negative impact on our health.

I must clarify a significant difference between the Natural Hygienic diet and modern "Raw Food" diets. Natural Hygiene advocates eating foods as they are grown in nature, without blending, juicing, dehydrating, fermenting, or processing. The focus is on simplicity and consuming foods in their natural state. On the other hand, modern raw foodists often create complex recipes with long ingredient lists, relying on appliances like blenders, juicers, and dehydrators for food preparation. They may also use numerous herbs and spices, adding a burden to the body that Natural Hygiene advises against. How we eat also matters - lengthy food preparation can strain our digestive system, while Natural Hygiene emphasizes the importance of simplicity and planning without the need for extensive processing. Building true health doesn't require hours of preparation, just a thoughtful approach to natural, whole foods.

The Pitfalls of Modern Raw Foodist and the Path to True Health

Over the course of my health journey and interactions with people, I've noticed an interesting pattern among modern "raw foodists." Many of them tend to indulge in heavier foods like nuts, seeds, avocados, and plant-based milks, believing these nutritionally dense foods are vital for sustenance. However, these high-fat and complex foods should ideally be consumed in moderation due to their difficulty in digestion and high protein/fat content.

Observing various dietary groups under the vegan umbrella, it becomes evident that some individuals rely heavily on these heavy foods as a substitute for the "substance" they were accustomed to in their past diets. This reliance leads to overconsumption of nuts, seeds, and fats, which can be detrimental to health over time. Arnold Ehret wisely taught that foods like avocado can be mucus-forming and thus should be limited in consumption.

In the raw food movement, nuts, seeds, and fats often become the main staples. Unfortunately, this overindulgence can lead to digestive issues, constipation, and other symptoms that eventually deter individuals from continuing the natural raw diet. It is crucial to strike a balance in the consumption of these nutritionally dense foods.

Humans are creatures of habit, and when transitioning to new dietary choices, it's common to fall into comfortable but potentially unhealthy habits. To achieve true healing, it is essential to simplify and transition properly to our species' appropriate diet, allowing time for adjustment. Many individuals are accustomed to eating until they feel full, but this habit must be overcome on the path to better health.

Overcoming overeating can be challenging, especially when dealing with the addictive nature of cooked and processed foods. However, as we align ourselves with our natural diet, we will naturally adjust our eating habits to meet our body's needs. Overeating places an unnecessary burden on the digestive system, depleting our life force energy and hindering overall health.

Transitioning to a natural diet involves understanding the proper balance of food choices and mindful eating practices. By respecting our body's needs and consuming the foods we are biologically designed for, we can restore our health and vitality, free from the burden of overconsumption and improper eating habits.

The Importance of a Proper Transition Diet

Embarking on a journey towards a healthier dietary regime is a significant step, and it is crucial to approach this transition with care and consideration. The concept of a proper "Transition Diet" plays a pivotal role in bridging the gap between a standard cooked food diet and a raw food or high raw diet, ensuring a smoother and more sustainable shift towards better health.

In the pursuit of a 100% raw food, plant-based diet, it is essential to recognize that this transition cannot happen overnight. For many individuals coming from generations of cooked food diets, such drastic changes may lead to setbacks and struggles if not undertaken thoughtfully and gradually.

Understanding the principles of the Transition Diet, as expounded by the renowned health pioneer Arnold Ehret in his book "The Mucusless Diet Healing System," serves as a foundational method to prepare our bodies for the return to our species' appropriate diet. The Transition Diet guides us on selecting less harmful foods from the cooked food kingdom that can be consumed while gradually transitioning to raw foods over time.

Ehret's teachings advocate the inclusion of steamed or baked vegetables in the Transition Diet. While Natural Hygiene promotes the consumption of raw plant fats in moderation, Ehret advises caution with overt plant fats due to their mucus-forming and constipating effects on the body. For instance, he recommends using lightly steamed vegetables as a source of satiety to help avoid harmful foods like mucus-forming avocados, nuts and seeds.

As individuals committed to a raw food diet, we can observe and experiment with our own bodies to understand what serves us best. The Transition Diet acts as a guide to make informed choices about the types of foods that can aid our journey towards optimal health.

When healing is the primary goal, it becomes essential to consume foods that require minimal digestive energy over extended periods. This approach allows the body to utilize its life force energy for healing and repair, rather than exhausting it in the complex digestion of heavy, difficult-to-digest foods.

The diet that fosters healing is the same diet that supports overall health and wellbeing. It is through simplicity and alignment with our natural dietary requirements that we can achieve lasting health benefits. The Transition Diet, in conjunction with a commitment to listening to our bodies and making informed choices, paves the way towards a vibrant and nourishing raw food lifestyle.

The Power of Whole Natural Foods in Transition

In our journey towards embracing a healthier lifestyle, we must not overlook the importance of consuming whole, natural foods in their unprocessed state. This principle is at the core of Natural Hygiene, a paradigm that encourages us to listen to our bodies and follow a diet that aligns with our natural design.

The transition from a standard cooked food diet to a raw food or high raw diet should be approached with mindful consideration. One aspect that often goes unnoticed in modern health circles is the significance of a proper "Transition Diet." This gradual shift helps our bodies adapt to healthier choices without overwhelming them and ensures a more sustainable path towards optimal health.

The world of juicing and smoothies may initially seem appealing, but it is vital to recognize that these practices process and alter the natural form of fruits and vegetables. By peeling and eating whole oranges, for instance, we allow our bodies to digest, absorb, assimilate, and eliminate the food as nature intended, preserving vital fiber and nutrients.

Natural Hygiene teaches us that our diet should consist of whole, natural foods until we feel satiated. This philosophy is the key to thriving, not merely surviving. It encourages us to focus on foods that form complete meals in their natural state, rather than relying on processed alternatives.

A distinction arises between the teachings of Natural

Hygiene and some modern raw foodists when it comes to the consumption of greens and fruits. Natural Hygiene places significant emphasis on eating greens, as it strengthens jaw and facial muscles, leading to strong, healthy teeth. Chewing greens unlocks essential nutrients that blending and juicing cannot provide.

Observing the raw food community, we find that some individuals tend to consume a plethora of raw vegetables and green juices while overlooking the role of healthy fruits. The fear of "sugar" leads to the avoidance of fruit consumption, resulting in digestive issues and the eventual abandonment of the raw food diet. In contrast, Natural Hygiene encourages a balanced approach, advocating the importance of fruits in our diet and promoting variety.

It is essential to distinguish between foods that are natural and beneficial for our bodies versus those that are not aligned with our true dietary requirements. Overindulgence in complex plant fats, fermented foods, and other raw but unnatural choices burdens the body, leading to health issues over time. Natural Hygiene promotes simplicity, steering us towards tender leafy greens, raw fruits, raw starchless vegetables, with minimal nuts, seeds, avocado, or plant fats.

Considering the Transition Diet recommended by Arnold Ehret, we find a focus on lightly steamed vegetables as a source of satiety during the shift towards a simple raw food diet. While Natural Hygiene views food from the perspective of burden on the body, Ehret emphasizes ease of elimination above all else. By incorporating steamed vegetables, he intended to aid the transition process and guide individuals towards a simpler raw food diet.

As we embrace the principles of Natural Hygiene, we learn to savor whole, natural foods and let go of the belief that abundance equals health. Listening to our bodies and consuming foods in their natural form empowers us to thrive and maintain a vibrant, nourished existence. By prioritizing simplicity and our species-appropriate diet, we unlock the path to true health and vitality.

Embracing the 100% Raw Journey

As I embarked on my 100% raw food journey, guided by the principles of Natural Hygiene after 8 years of transitioning, I felt a sense of determination and excitement. My commitment to this lifestyle was driven by a desire to truly understand the impact of this dietary choice on my body and well-being. Having followed The Mucusless Diet Healing System for several years, I knew that I was a prime candidate for this experiment.

My plan was simple yet profound. I decided to dedicate a minimum of six months to this endeavor, with minimal nuts and seeds. This approach allowed me to gauge the impact of Hygienic principles on my body, comparing it to the time when I consumed steamed vegetables instead of plant fats.

Adopting a 100% raw food diet felt like a natural progression for me, considering my diet had already been about 80-90% raw for over eight years. The transition was surprisingly seamless, as the most time-consuming aspect of my previous food preparation had been steaming or baking vegetables without condiments, oil, spices, or salts of any kind.

Engaging with Natural Hygienic studies taught me invaluable lessons about health and disease. I learned that unlearning the misinformation we were taught over the years is a significant challenge. Our species has strayed so far from our natural diet and lifestyle that the truth on how to live healthily can seem absurd. However, the simplicity and logic of the Natural Hygiene approach resonates with me deeply.

I have observed that people's motivation to change their dietary habits often stems from the suffering caused by major health issues. Unfortunately, society tends to normalize suffering as part of the aging process, accepting it as "normal." However, healthy decisions stem from healthy individuals, and I firmly believe that a healthy population can create a better world.

One aspect of the raw food community that caught my attention was the overconsumption of certain raw foods that are not natural for us to eat. Some individuals eat fermented foods, raw oils, and processed raw products, often driven by the belief that if it is raw, it is healthy. In contrast, Natural Hygiene emphasizes simplicity and focuses on tender leafy greens, raw fruits, and raw starchless vegetables with minimal nuts, seeds, avocado, or plant fats.

During my 100% raw journey, I discovered that overindulgence in plant fats can burden the body. Therefore, I adopted a cautious approach and used nuts and seeds sparingly, primarily for salad dressings. The careful balance of my diet allowed me to maintain vitality and avoid the digestive discomfort associated with overindulgence.

My experience reinforced my belief that learning the truth about our species-appropriate diet is vital. While not everyone may choose to follow it entirely, having the knowledge empowers individuals to make informed decisions about their health.

As my six-month journey came to an end, I felt a deep sense of contentment. The experiment had taught me valuable insights, and I was ready to continue my optimal health lifestyle. Armed with the wisdom of Natural Hygiene, I moved forward, grateful to all those who preserved and passed on this life-changing information. The journey may be ongoing, but with every step, I find myself closer to living a life of vibrant health and vitality.

Update: I completed the 6 months 100% raw keeping my overt fat intake to roughly around 10% of my daily dietary intake. The purpose of making a point about this is that I want to find out once and for all what is more of a burden on the body, the steamed vegetables or the plant fats (assuming you had to pick one or the other) and to be honest, if I keep the plant fats low, I do not feel much of a difference between the two. If I overdo fats at all, the next day I can feel it. I will feel tired, bloated, sluggish and have a bit of a food hangover. If I overdo steamed vegetables, I do not feel the same burden as overdoing the plant fats, however, I will feel a bit bloated, but it seems the symptoms are less. This doesn't mean that I am turning back to including steamed vegetables in my diet because I feel good keeping everything raw and not cooking at all. I just want to know for information purposes, and I will continue my quest to find out which is more of a burden on the body, lightly steamed vegetables, or consuming plant fats. That is all for this chapter, thanks for taking the time to read through my thoughts and experiences.

Chapter 8
Dr. Joel Fuhrman, M.D.

Dr. Joel Fuhrman, M.D., is a highly esteemed figure in the field of nutrition and natural healing. As an American board-certified family physician, bestselling author, and expert in nutrition, he has dedicated his career to helping individuals overcome health issues and reverse chronic diseases using dietary interventions. His focus lies in tackling conditions like obesity, diabetes, heart disease, and other chronic ailments through the power of nutrition.

One of Dr. Fuhrman's notable contributions to health education is his development of the "**G-Bombs**" acronym. This acronym serves as a simplified guide to his dietary recommendations, making it easier for individuals to remember and apply the principles of his optimal diet.

With six New York Times bestsellers to his credit, Dr. Fuhrman's books have reached and influenced a wide audience, providing valuable insights into improving health and well-being through proper nutrition. Titles like "Eat to Live," "Fast Food Genocide," and "Eat for Life" have become well-known resources in the pursuit of a healthier lifestyle.

Dr. Fuhrman's approach to healing and health emphasizes the power of natural foods and their potential to positively impact our well-being. His expertise, scientific knowledge, and commitment to sharing the benefits of plant-based nutrition have earned him recognition and respect in the medical and health community.

As a specialist in reversing chronic diseases, Dr. Joel Fuhrman's work has had a profound impact on countless lives, empowering individuals to take charge of their health and make positive changes through dietary choices. His contribution to the field of nutrition and natural healing continues to inspire people worldwide to embrace healthier habits and pursue a disease-free life.

Dr. Joel Fuhrman's commitment to helping people achieve optimal health extends beyond his books and online resources. Through the "Eat to Live" retreat center in the picturesque hills of San Diego, he offers a more intimate and interactive setting to assist individuals in building healthier, long-term dietary and lifestyle habits. He works with individuals in small, interactive settings, where he can provide personalized assistance in building healthier and sustainable lifestyle habits. At his retreat, organic plant-based meals, including fresh vegetables from their own garden, are served, creating a nurturing environment for learning and transformation.

At the retreat center, Dr. Fuhrman personally works with patients, providing one-on-one guidance and support. This personalized approach allows him to better understand everyone's specific health needs and tailor his recommendations accordingly.

The retreat center experience typically spans three weeks to a month, giving participants ample time to immerse themselves in Dr. Fuhrman's nutritional approach. The longer duration ensures that attendees gain a thorough knowledge base and practical experience, enabling them to integrate his recommendations into their daily lives even after they leave the retreat.

The retreat's emphasis on organic, plant-based meals underscores Dr. Fuhrman's commitment to providing the most nourishing and healthy foods. The inclusion of fresh vegetables from the retreat's garden further highlights the focus on whole, nutrient-dense foods.

In addition to the nourishing meals, Dr. Fuhrman offers a comprehensive educational program during the retreat. Through lectures, educational talks, and informative sessions, attendees gain an in-depth understanding of the principles behind his nutritional approach. This knowledge equips them to make informed choices and confidently incorporate the healthful habits they've learned into their daily routines beyond the retreat.

I included Dr. Joel Fuhrman among my list of health practitioners because I truly resonate with his approach to nutrition and natural healing. As a board-certified family physician and best-selling author, Dr. Fuhrman focuses on using nutrition to reverse various chronic diseases like obesity, diabetes, and heart disease.

His emphasis on nutrient density and overall health aligns with my personal beliefs.

Listening to countless YouTube videos of Dr. Fuhrman's health discussions over the years, I can genuinely feel his passion for helping people achieve a disease-free life filled with vitality. His practical approach to dietary recommendations, such as the "G-Bombs" acronym, simplifies healthy eating choices, making it easier to remember and follow.

Dr. Fuhrman's emphasis on staying at the retreat for a minimum of 3 weeks to a month ensures that participants have the necessary knowledge and experience to apply his recommendations long-term. The combination of informative lectures, educational talks, and practical guidance helps individuals understand how to incorporate these healthful habits into their real-world lives effectively.

Personally, I find his advice on daily greens, especially in the form of a large-sized salad, to be particularly resonating. His balanced approach to caloric intake, warning against both overeating and undereating, makes sense and helps maintain a healthy balance.

While I greatly respect the insights of classic authors like Herbert Shelton, Arnold Ehret, and TC Fry, I understand that some people prefer information from more contemporary sources. Dr. Fuhrman's approach bridges the gap, offering modern insights that can be easily embraced by those looking to improve their health without committing to a 100% raw food diet.

As I continue writing my book, I aim to provide a valuable resource that blends time-tested wisdom with up-to-date insights. I want to share information that helps people make informed choices about their health and well-being, catering to a wide range of preferences and needs. Recommending Dr. Joel Fuhrman is part of my commitment to offering holistic and accessible health advice to all.

Dr. Joel Fuhrman's dietary recommendations revolve around achieving "Nutritional Excellence" for optimal health and the prevention and reversal of diseases. His primary emphasis is on a nutrient-rich, plant-based diet. Dr. Fuhrman advises against the consumption of animal products, but he understands that some individuals may not be ready to give up meat completely. In such cases, he suggests reducing animal product intake and focusing primarily on incorporating healthy plant foods into the diet.

One of the core principles of Dr. Fuhrman's approach is adopting an **SOS-free diet**, which means avoiding added **s**alt, **o**il, and **s**ugar. Many health circles are now recognizing the adverse effects of processed oils and salt on health, making this recommendation increasingly popular.

The acronym "**G-Bombs**" coined by Dr. Fuhrman represents the most health-promoting superfoods: "**G**reens", "**B**eans", "**O**nions", "**M**ushrooms", "**B**erries", and "**S**eeds". He advocates including these nutrient-dense foods in the daily diet to promote overall well-being.

His "**G-Bombs**" acronym resonates with me, especially the "**G**reens" part. I wholeheartedly agree that incorporating a large leafy green salad daily is essential for our health. In my own experience, a daily salad has been instrumental in maintaining healthy teeth, strong jaw muscles, and regular bowel movements.

I also support the idea of using **B**eans as a transition food for those eliminating animal products from their diet. While Beans are complex and high in protein, they are less burdensome on the digestive system compared to meat and animal products. However, I suggest using Beans temporarily, as they are not part of our long-term species-appropriate diet.

Regarding Dr. Fuhrman's recommendation for **O**nions, I respectfully disagree. Onions are irritants and can cause damage to the digestive organs. I believe they are not fit for human consumption, as suggested by Natural Hygiene principles. I have personally experienced the negative effects of consuming onions and garlic, leading me to eliminate them from my diet.

As for **M**ushrooms, they can serve as satisfying transition foods, especially in replacing meat in certain dishes. I agree that they are better alternatives to processed vegan meat replacers, as they do not contain additives and preservatives.

The recommendation for **B**erries is excellent, as they provide healthy sugars that are essential for our bodies. However, I encourage including a variety of fruits in the diet, not just berries. Dr. Fuhrman's advice to eat fruit fresh and avoid processed fruit products aligns with my beliefs as well.

When it comes to **S**eeds, I advocate moderation. While they are part of a healthy human diet, consuming them daily can be excessive. I keep my plant fats intake, including nuts and seeds, to around 10% of my daily intake. It is essential not to overdo fats and to avoid combining them with sugars in the same meal for proper digestion.

Overall, I find Dr. Fuhrman's dietary recommendations to be a valuable resource for those seeking a healthier diet. Although I may not agree with all aspects, I appreciate that he provides a bridge between a standard diet and a healthier plant-based one. It's encouraging to see medical doctors like him promoting plant-based diets for improved health, as their recommendations can be influential for those seeking medical advice.

In addition to dietary recommendations, Dr. Fuhrman believes in the potential benefits of supplements to address potential nutrient deficiencies or insufficiencies that some individuals may experience. As discussed in previous chapters, I believe that supplements are not the answer and only serve to suppress symptoms which does not address the root cause.

On his website, "www.drfuhrman.com", you can find scientific studies, informative videos, details about his health retreat, recipes, and more, all aimed at guiding individuals towards better health and nutritional knowledge.

Chapter 9
Dealing with Headaches and Unwanted Symptoms

Over the course of many years, I worked to resolve my recurring headaches. While I successfully addressed various health issues, these headaches remained a persistent challenge. They were the last symptom I needed to overcome, and it took a considerable effort to find a remedy. I've dedicated a whole chapter to this topic because the insights I gained were truly enlightening.

Most, if not all, of our symptoms are signals of internal toxicity. Our current dietary and lifestyle habits often don't align with our body's true needs, unless the symptoms stem from detoxification due to healthier dietary changes or trauma such as accidents. Inflammation manifests in numerous ways, or rather, through various symptoms.

I've discussed my lifelong journey dealing with worsening symptoms, with the most distressing being the recurring, intense headaches that started in my late teens and persisted into my 30s. If given a choice, I'd opt for almost any pain over a headache (except for tooth pain). In the past, I managed these unbearable headaches and other pains with various pharmaceutical painkillers, using them regularly to prevent morning headaches. Unaware of the long-term consequences, I numbed my nervous system to suppress symptoms. Little did I know this would contribute to internal toxicity and liver damage down the road.

When I discovered a path to healing my health issues, my anticipation of becoming headache-free was a driving force. Within two years of adopting a vegan, high-fruit diet and eliminating meats, animal products, and unhealthy items like eggs, chocolate, and wine, most of my health problems improved. This progress motivated me to continue this dietary approach as a long-term lifestyle, rather than an experiment.

After roughly five years on this healthful journey, I realized that although I had resolved most of my symptoms, I still experienced occasional headaches every couple of months. These headaches were less severe compared to the past, but I questioned why they persisted after so long on a healthy path. I wanted to heal them completely, as they were a reminder of past suffering and an obstacle to feeling my best.

Eventually, I made the breakthrough. After reading a short book, "Correct Living or The Fountain of Happiness" by Van R. Wilcox, written in 1906, I discovered the missing piece to my health puzzle. This book, which was sent to me by an acquaintance on Facebook, turned out to be transformative. Its insights resonated with me at the right time, when I was prepared to take the necessary steps to finally heal my headache issues.

There are a few key points that I read throughout those pages that I will share in my own words. According to Van R. Wilcox, the process of stomach digestion essentially stops while we sleep, rendering large or any meals (apart from fruit, which digests in 2-5 hours) to sit undigested in the stomach during the night. This stagnant food, when combined with body heat, undergoes decomposition and fermentation, causing the loss of energy from a significant portion of the consumed food. This process becomes worse due to the creation of poisonous substances because of the decomposition and fermentation, which are absorbed into the bloodstream, leading to various symptoms such as bad breath, headaches, rheumatism, and colds. Van R. Wilcox asserts that this phenomenon is a primary trigger for our health problems.

Furthermore, Wilcox explains that the situation worsens in the morning when breakfast is consumed, adding to the ongoing fermentation. This is followed by another large meal a few hours later, and then dinner, all of which contribute to gas production and discomfort. Wilcox advocates for the "No Breakfast Plan," aligning with Professor Arnold Ehret's perspective. Ehret might have drawn inspiration from Wilcox's book "Correct Living," considering it was written before Ehret's time and both authors used the "No Breakfast Plan" terminology. It's worth noting that I had already eliminated breakfast from my routine years ago, especially as one of the initial adjustments following Arnold Ehret's teachings. For more than 9 years, my first meal of the day has consistently begun with juicy fruits.

Around the seven-year mark of my health journey, I delved deeper into Natural Hygiene and discovered a correlation with

Van R. Wilcox's insights. Natural Hygiene emphasizes three 8-hour cycles of the body within a day: from noon to 8 pm, optimal digestion occurs; from 8 pm to 4 am, assimilation takes place; and from 4 am to noon, elimination or cleansing mode is active. This aligns with Wilcox's idea of undigested food remaining in the stomach during rest. Hence, it's crucial to avoid eating at least 1-2 hours before sleep or before 8 pm.

Now, let's look at another aspect of the headache and unexplained symptom puzzle. This aspect, which I'll call the "Elephant in the Room," sheds light on why many "vegans" or "plant-based" individuals struggle and eventually revert back to meat-based or harmful diets. It's an often ignored but significant factor critical for a healthy body and life. This aspect is frequently underestimated because it appears minor, making it challenging for most people to address Overeating.

How much is too much?

In the various vegan Facebook groups that I'm a part of, a common sentiment prevails: if you're on a plant-based diet—whether cooked or raw, fruits or healthy plant-based foods—you can eat as much as you want. I admit I've fallen into this mindset, and it's a mindset that has contributed to my recurring headaches. I wanted to believe it was true. For around 7 years, my main meal of the day was an extensive evening salad topped with raw or lightly steamed vegetables and dressing usually composed of raw or cooked tomato sauce, avocado, or tahini. I would eat until I was uncomfortably full, almost bloated. My salad portion was akin to what a typical family of four might share, a size that wouldn't be an issue if all my food were 100% raw. However, this wasn't the case.

I sought that sensation of fullness to suppress my stress and emotions, a common coping mechanism. I justified this behavior by assuming that since the foods were less calorie dense and simple, overeating wasn't a significant concern. It felt like I needed to stuff myself in this lifestyle, consuming more than necessary. Part of this was linked to past dietary habits, with the stored waste from those choices playing a role.

To clarify, I always intuitively understood that overeating wasn't ideal, but I didn't fully grasp its detrimental impact on overall health. I attempted to eat smaller meals on several occasions, but it seemed unattainable, leading me to give up. It's worth noting that during the initial transition from an animal-based diet to a plant-based one, overeating is common. Over time, the urge to overeat subsides, but during those initial years, it's important to be aware of this tendency and work towards moderation.

Overeating often stems from compensating for previous diets rich in complex foods. This inclination diminishes over time as we heal and come into alignment, but understanding the process is essential. Overeating can also arise to suppress uncomfortable elimination symptoms triggered by the body. Failing to confront these symptoms and the discomfort they bring can lead to a vicious cycle that only ends when we take a proactive approach.

Van R. Wilcox and Arnold Ehret both emphasized that foul body odors, including bad breath, can only originate from internal filth. Ehret discussed how overeating creates a "cesspool" in the stomach. This excess food ferments, decays, and putrefies, polluting the entire body. This contamination affects not only breath but also flesh and blood, which becomes poisoned. It's intriguing because during a past headache, I had described the feeling as if I had been poisoned, a sentiment that resonates with these teachings.

Wilcox explained that blood circulates through the stomach walls with every heartbeat, absorbing its contents, whether "good or evil." Properly treating food through chewing and consuming a reasonable amount prevents decay and putrefaction, ensuring proper digestion and nutrient absorption for blood circulation to build the body as intended. He asserted that by eating reasonably and chewing food to a liquid form, over time, issues like headaches, constipation, joint discomfort, skin problems, and more can be eliminated.

This information was captivating because, despite having a seemingly correct and health-promoting diet, I sensed there were missing pieces to the health puzzle. Reading Wilcox's book filled in those gaps. To rid myself of headaches, I needed to eat smaller, yet substantial meals and thoroughly chew my food. Sometimes, the small but crucial aspects are overlooked and hold immense significance.

As for conquering overeating, an interesting shift occurred. I decided to slightly modify my diet by introducing starches and eliminating fats entirely, a change to my existing routine of raw fruits, greens, and raw/steamed vegetables. I embarked on Dr. John McDougall's "Starch Solution Diet" for a 100-day trial to speak from personal experience and verify its efficacy. However, after 75 days, I felt the decline in my well-being, including negative moods and reduced vitality, which prompted me to abandon the experiment early.

Quitting the starch-based diet coincided with an excruciating 8-day headache. This experience became a turning point. Something within me shifted; I had reached a point of enough. Pain proved to be an influential motivator. I made changes because I couldn't bear the prospect of recurring headaches. This time, the attempt to eat smaller meals succeeded remarkably, unlike my previous struggles. I felt as if I had hit rock bottom and had no choice but to adapt. I began chewing all my food to a liquid before swallowing, which demanded patience and time. Surprisingly, I no longer desired large meals but instead craved simple foods like fruits, plain vegetables, and greens.

Chewing food properly is a crucial but often underestimated aspect of a healthy diet. Despite the common belief that the stomach breaks down food, insufficient chewing can lead to suboptimal functioning of our "human machine." This practice tends to be overlooked and under-addressed in the health community, which is unfortunate because thoroughly chewing food to a liquid form could potentially resolve numerous health issues. Although most people are aware of the importance of proper chewing, distractions and lack of focus often prevent its consistent implementation.

By thoroughly chewing food to liquid form before swallowing, overeating became impossible. I've been consuming half the amount I used to during meals, feeling more satisfied. I learned that much of digestion occurs in the mouth, and proper chewing aids nutrient absorption. This practice has significantly improved my overall well-being, underscoring the importance of optimal digestion, assimilation, and absorption through thorough chewing.

To chew every bite into a liquid requires being present and

focused on the meal, free from distractions. My initial days of proper chewing left my jaw sore, a clear sign of how little I had been chewing before. Around day five of smaller meals combined with proper chewing, I experienced a day of sickness. Despite rarely falling ill, I recognized this as part of my body's re-adjustment and detoxification process. During this episode, I rested, fasted on water, and recovered in a day, reaffirming the importance of rest during sickness.

It's important to clarify that I now eat until I'm satisfied instead of overeating. Since transitioning to a 100% raw diet, I've noticed I can eat more comfortably than when I included cooked foods. Cooked food's addictive and stimulating nature often leads to overeating. Raw foods, on the other hand, lack the same urge to overconsume. While it's true that our species is designed for eating volume, it's essential to consume the right foods. Otherwise, volume can easily translate into overeating and fermentation issues.

Creating a new habit like proper chewing takes time, trial, and error. To remind myself, I set daily cellphone reminders and even explored literature like "Fletcherism" by Horace Fletcher, which emphasizes chewing properly. Although I appreciated its insights into mouth digestion, I was disappointed by the lack of awareness regarding ideal dietary requirements for humans. As a result, I didn't finish the book.

As I write this, it has been close to a year since I abandoned the Starch Solution Diet and began thoroughly chewing my food before swallowing. The impact of this practice has been truly remarkable. Proper chewing has become a habitual part of my routine, and I'm surprised it took me so long to adopt such a beneficial habit. My nighttime rest has improved. I opt for a light evening meal, usually a good sized raw salad, as it's easier for the body to digest. My largest meal, which includes fruit, is consumed during the daytime (12-2pm) to allow for proper digestion – a process that has been significantly enhanced by my diligent chewing.

The positive changes have been numerous: my digestion has improved, headaches have ceased, and my mood and thoughts are consistently positive. I'm immensely proud of myself for overcoming my last dietary and health hurdle, finally completing this puzzle. The discomfort I experienced while attempting the Starch Solution Diet, combined with overeating and improper chewing, acted as a strong motivation to refine my habits. This might sound peculiar, but feeling chronically unwell each day is a powerful incentive for change. Having already come so far from a past of constant discomfort, I'm determined never to return to that state.

Health is the foundation of a fulfilling life. Without it, life's potential is limited, and we can't achieve what we're truly capable of. The pain I endured during my experience with the Starch Solution Diet, combined with overeating and inadequate chewing, served as a forceful catalyst for change. Sometimes, suffering serves as a wake-up call. Having successfully overcome major health issues in the past, I knew what steps to take to restore my well-being. I refuse to go back to the days of frequent headaches, aches, and unexplained symptoms. My journey has brought me too far to regress.

Gratitude extends to myself and to all the authors, healers, and insightful individuals from whom I've gained invaluable knowledge. Their contributions have paved the way for my healing journey. I'm also appreciative of those who shared books and gifts as a gesture of reciprocity for the helpful information I've shared. It's heartening to know that achieving optimal health is a choice accessible to most people. Learning and taking necessary steps toward healing are within reach.

Stay Hydrated

Now, for arguably the most significant aspect of solving the headache issue – a point that I've saved for last and that anyone can incorporate immediately, regardless of their diet. In fact, I highly recommend implementing this solution without delay, no matter your dietary choices. Headaches stem from pollution circulating in the bloodstream, indicating toxicity. I came across a phrase, *"The Solution for Pollution IS Dilution,"* coined by Lauren Whiteman, which holds invaluable wisdom. To address the acids causing headaches, we must dilute them by drinking more water, ideally distilled. Drinking a gallon of water a day (or even 1.5 gallons) can lead to a noticeable reduction or complete elimination of headaches over time.

It's important to note that there are no quick fixes. Unlike pharmaceuticals that merely suppress symptoms, proper hydration requires time. For over a year now, I've consistently consumed about 3-4 liters of water daily, resulting in enhanced well-being. However, the goal is to reach a gallon a day consistently by June of this year, a gradual process that requires time and adjustment. This transition was particularly challenging for me due to a lifelong aversion to water. I'd hardly drink more than a couple of glasses a day, if that. This chronic dehydration, compounded by a predominantly dehydrating diet, contributed to my past symptoms.

Furthermore, if we overeat or consume foods outside our species-appropriate diet, fermentation may occur, leading to less-than-ideal blood content. In my case, I believe inadequate hydration played a crucial role in the persistence of my headaches. Most of us, like me, have dealt with chronic dehydration from childhood onward, failing to compensate for our dehydrating diets. Even the commonly recommended 8 glasses of water a day fall short when combating dehydration caused by less-than-ideal dietary choices. To fully compensate, we need to drink 1-1.5 gallons of water daily. It's worth reflecting on the fact that our species-appropriate diet consists of water-rich foods like fruits, greens, some vegetables, and minimal nuts/seeds, completely devoid of dehydrating elements.

The notion of writing a book has been a lifelong aspiration of mine, rooted in a childhood belief that someday I would become an author, even though the purpose behind it remained unclear. Looking back, it's evident that I lacked the essential information needed to express what I had to offer until now, explaining the lengthy process. I am now confident that I have unraveled the enigma surrounding my health and am preparing to finalize this chapter before sending it for publication, reaffirming the complete resolution of my headaches. This achievement resulted from my willingness to modify my habits when new insights emerged.

Update:

As of January 18, 2023, I am proud to announce a continued absence of headaches. Progress sometimes entails taking a few steps backward to propel oneself forward, a principle I embraced wholeheartedly to ensure comprehensive validation. My decision to adopt a 100% vegan lifestyle by eliminating animal products and meats remains pivotal. This initial step towards reclaiming my health has instilled a profound sense of gratitude within me. Despite numerous attempts over the years by well-meaning individuals to sway my dietary choices, I remain resolute in abstaining from foods I consider detrimental to human well-being. The adverse impact of such items on health is something I am deeply acquainted with, and I am unwavering in my commitment to never revert to the days of experiencing debilitating headaches. My journey has come too far, and I place the utmost value on well-being, recognizing its role as a foundation for meaningful service to others.

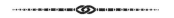

Chapter 10
The Mucusless Diet Healing System Food Lists

Within this chapter, I'll provide you with comprehensive lists of foods that align with a wholesome and natural human diet, as well as foods that have the potential to induce mucus formation and acidity in the body.

I am excited to present to you the "revised transcript" of the original "Berg's tables", carefully compiled by the knowledgeable Professor Spira. These tables were originally featured in Arnold Ehret's timeless book, "The Mucusless Diet Healing System". However, in order to eliminate any confusion for first time readers, Professor Spira took the liberty to make valuable editorial amendments which was originally featured in his "ANNOTATED EDITION of the MUCUSLESS DIET". The intent with this revised transcript is to provide you with a clearer understanding of the concepts that were previously conveyed in the original somewhat confusing "Berg's tables". Professor Spira's expert annotations have enhanced and improved the text, making it easier to understand for everyone For a deeper understanding and practical implementation of the «Mucusless Diet Healing System» in your lifestyle, I strongly recommend reading Professor Spira's book titled "PROF. ARNOLD EHRET'S MUCUSLESS DIET HEALING SYSTEM ANNOTATED, REVISED, AND EDITED BY PROF. SPIRA", or the Original Arnold Ehret's books, "The Mucusless Diet Healing System" and "Rational Fasting." Personally, I've followed the Mucusless Diet Healing System for over 9 years, and I can confidently assert that no other system I know of compares to Ehret's methods and information on transitioning from a standard diet to a healthy plant-based, high-fruit diet. This approach isn't merely a diet but a system and lifestyle that can benefit anyone, regardless of their current stage, by enhancing their health.

Ehret›s teachings provide a fundamental understanding of our genuine dietary needs, guiding us to bridge the gap between past unhealthy eating habits and healthier choices. His work, from the early 1900s, offers unique insights not commonly found in today›s health profession. Thanks to a few dedicated individuals sharing his work such as Professor Spira, his knowledge remains relevant to this day.

In our contemporary world, simplicity is the essence of truth, while complexity pervades every aspect. The confusion around what to eat and how to nourish ourselves leads many to attempt fad diets only to give up. To discern truth, I adhere to a simple rule: listen to those who have achieved the results you seek. The Mucusless Diet Healing System enables us to understand optimal foods for human health, and its effectiveness can be easily verified through a fair trial. Once we experience the healing and witness our most distressing symptoms subside, the motivation to continue this transformative journey becomes self-evident.

Rebuilding our health transcends dietary changes; it necessitates addressing various life aspects for holistic well-being. A comprehensive grasp of Arnold Ehret›s system, combined with practical application, empowers us to make well-informed decisions in any situation. It›s imperative to not overlook the depth of Ehret›s teachings – a common mistake made by those who merely skim his food lists. To gain the full benefit, delve into his books. Fortunately, a wide variety of the healthiest foods from fruit, vegetable, and leafy green realms are accessible globally. I look forward to someday traveling the world, sampling diverse fruits and raw foods.

Transitioning entails using some cooked vegetables and fruits as transitional foods to satisfy cravings and aid in eliminating accumulated waste. Ehret›s recommendations encompass more than just fruits and raw, mucusless foods. He's devised a system for gradual, safe transitions to healthier dietary and lifestyle habits. Incorporating foods like starchless steamed vegetables with a generous green salad can act as an intestinal broom, facilitating waste elimination. A salad when paired with other less-than-ideal foods enhances digestion and elimination.

When cravings arise, Mucusless Diet practitioners opt for cooked, starchless vegetables over fatty foods like nuts and seeds – choices that align with Ehret›s principles. While I›ve experimented with both approaches, discerning which burdens the body less remains challenging. Ehret advised limiting plant fats, ideally consuming them sparingly during winter months. Determining the lesser burden between plant fats and steamed vegetables is essential. My personal journey from a high raw to an exclusively raw diet unfolded over 7 years, making the transition more manageable. Patience and understanding are vital during this process.

Arnold Ehret›s teachings offer unique insights not found elsewhere. He emphasizes not only what we eat but how we consume it, impacting the mucus-forming properties of foods. For example, poached or fried eggs are more mucus-forming than hard-boiled eggs. Baking certain foods, like potatoes, can reduce mucus formation. While I don›t advocate eating such foods, Ehret›s insights help mitigate harm for those transitioning. When consuming less than ideal foods, like bread, toasting can minimize mucus-forming properties.

Healing from years of consuming mucus-forming foods takes time. Rapid changes or extremes can lead to unforeseen issues. It›s important to embark on a gradual transition, building sustainable habits. Bioaccumulation underlies our health woes, and diseases represent the body›s efforts to expel accumulated waste. Symptoms indicate the curative process; interfering with it hinders healing. Rest, hydration, fresh air, patience, and understanding are the body›s true needs during this phase. Patience is key; nature doesn›t rush healing.

Ultimately, the journey toward optimal health involves much more than dietary changes. It demands a comprehensive approach and a commitment to gradual, lasting transformation. Feel free to reference the Mucusless food lists to remind yourself that our present symptoms are outcomes of past choices. Amidst today›s conflicting health information, it›s easy to lose sight of the truth. Nature›s slow pace guides healing, and patience, coupled with proper understanding, makes the journey easier. The body knows how to heal itself; our role is to facilitate its processes by reducing burdens and allowing it the rest it requires.

To begin, let's categorize the Mucusless Foods, which fall under the Fruit, Vegetable, and Leafy Green Kingdom. These foods are non-obstructive to the body's functioning and undergo easy digestion, demanding minimal energy. They align with our species' inherent dietary needs, devoid of disease-promoting properties.

Nurturing an awareness of mucusless foods is crucial, emphasizing that fruits should be fully ripe and consumed in their natural state to foster optimal health.

Here is a comprehensive list of mucusless foods from the Fruit Kingdom:

- Apples

- Apricots

- Bananas

- Berries (including blueberries, strawberries, raspberries, etc.)

- Black Cherries (all varieties of cherries)

- Oranges

- Cantaloupe

- Grapefruit

- Grapes

- Honeydew

- Kiwi

- Lemons

- Limes

- Mandarin Oranges

- Mangoes

- Nectarines

- Peaches

- Pears

- Pineapple

- Plums

- Pomegranates

- Prunes

- Raisins

- Strawberries

- Tangerines

- Watermelon

 Incorporating these fruits into your diet can contribute to improved health, as they align with our natural dietary requirements and promote ease of digestion. Remember, opting for ripe and unprocessed forms of these fruits is key to harnessing their full health benefits.

Additionally, dried and baked fruits also fall within the realm of mucusless foods, though they are not as optimal as fresh alternatives. It's crucial to understand that the drying process removes water from these foods, making it essential to maintain proper hydration by consuming adequate water, ideally about half an hour before consuming dried fruits.

Here is a list of mucusless dried and baked fruits:

- Apples

- Apricots

- Bananas

- Blueberries

- Cherries

- Cranberries

- Currants

- Dates (both dried and fresh)

- Figs (both dried and fresh)

- Grapes (both dried/raisins and fresh)

- Kiwi

- Mango

- Peach

- Pears

- Pineapple

- Plums/Prunes

- Strawberries

While not as ideal as their fresh counterparts, these dried and baked fruits are still healthier options compared to many other cooked foods. Just remember to prioritize water intake, particularly before consuming dried fruits, due to their reduced water content. Incorporating these choices into your diet can contribute to your overall health and well-being.

Within the category of "Slightly Mucus-Forming" foods, you can find starchy or fatty vegetables and fruits. It's important to note that while these foods are not as mucus-forming as others, they still possess some mild mucus-forming potential. Here is a list of these foods:

- Artichoke

- Avocados

- Carrots (Raw)

- Cassava

- Cauliflower (Raw)

- Coconut Meat

- Corn

- Durian

- Green Peas

- Mushrooms (Fungus)

- Olives

- Onions

- Parsnips

- Peas (Raw)

- Plantains

- Pumpkin

- White Potato (Raw or Baked)

- Sweet Potato (Raw)

- Rutabaga

- Squash (Raw)

- Turnip

- Unripe Banana

- Winter Acorn Squash (Raw)

- Winter Butternut (Raw)

- All Winter Squashes (Raw)

These foods possess a level of mucus-forming potential but are still healthier options compared to other cooked or processed foods. Balancing their consumption with a variety of mucusless and less mucus-forming options can contribute to a more healthful diet.

Now, let's explore the world of greens and the various types of vegetables that fall under the category of Acid-Binding, Non-Mucus-Forming, or Mucusless (Mucus Free Foods). It's important to acknowledge that there can be discrepancies between different teachings, such as Natural Hygiene and Arnold Ehret's recommendations. Individual experience and judgment play a role in deciding what works best for each person.

Here's a breakdown of the greens and other vegetables that align with the concept of mucusless or non-mucus-forming foods:

**Green Leaf Vegetables (Considered "Mucusless") **:

- Arugula

- Bok Choi

- Cabbage

- Dandelion Leaf

- Greens (Kale, Mustard, Turnip, Collards, etc.)

- Leafy Herbs (Basil, Parsley, Cilantro, Rosemary, Thyme, etc.)

- Lettuce (Green, Red, Romaine, Boston Bibb, Iceberg, etc.)

- Spinach

- Swiss Chard

- Watercress

**Raw Vegetables/Root, Stem, Fruits (Relatively "Starchless" or "Mucusless") **:

- Asparagus

- Black Radish

- Broccoli

- Brussels Sprouts

- Celery

- Cucumbers

- Dandelion

- Dill

- Endives

- Green Onions

- Horse Radish

- Leeks

- Peppers (Green, Red, Yellow, Orange)

- Red Beets

- Red Cabbage

- Rhubarb

- Sea Vegetables

- Sugar Beets

- Tomatoes

- Young Radish

- Zucchini

**Baked Vegetables / Root, Stem, Fruits (Relatively "Starchless" or "Mucusless") **:

- Acorn Squash (Baked)

- Asparagus

- Broccoli (Steamed or Baked)

- Brussels Sprouts (Steamed)

- Butternut Squash (Baked)

- Carrots (Steamed)

- Cauliflower (Steamed or Baked)

- Green Peas (Steamed)

- Peppers (Green, Red, Yellow, Orange)

- Pumpkins (Steamed or Baked)

- Spaghetti Squash (Baked)

- Sweet Potato (Baked)

- Zucchini (Steamed or Baked)

These vegetables contribute to a diet rich in non-mucus-forming options, aligning with the principles of mucusless eating. Balancing these choices with other mucusless and less mucus-forming foods can aid in promoting overall health and well-being. Remember, individual preferences and responses play a role in determining which foods work best for you.

Here is a list of sweeteners that are generally considered mucusless if they are preservative-free:

- Agave Nectar

- Fruit Jellies with no artificial sugars added

- Maple Syrup

- Molasses

- Honey

These sweeteners, when devoid of artificial additives and preservatives, can be incorporated into a mucusless diet. Remember to use them in moderation, as excessive consumption of any sweeteners can affect overall health.

Animal Products - Pus Forming:

- All animal flesh (chicken, beef, goat, horse, dog, lamb, etc.)

- Animal blood

- Pork (bacon, ham, sausage, pigs' feet, etc.)

- Turkey

- Veal

- Wild Game (buffalo, bison, rabbit, deer, birds, venison, ostrich, etc.)

Seafood - Pus Forming:

- Fish

- Crab

- Crayfish

- Lobster

- Shrimp

- Caviar

- Salmon

- Shellfish

- Oysters

- Clams

- All seafood

Dairy Products - Pus Forming:

- All butter

- Buttermilk

- Cheese (all types)

- Cream

- Eggs (hard-boiled, scrambled, yolk, whites)

- Lard

- Margarine

- Goat milk

- Sheep milk

- Cow milk

- Skim milk

- Yogurt

**Moderately Mucus Forming Foods (Avoid when Striving for Optimal Health) **:

- Barley

- Bread (all types)

- Buckwheat

- Cornmeal

- Farina

- Kamut

- Macaroni

- Millet

- Oats

- Pastas (wheat, rice, corn, etc.)

- White rice

- Quinoa

- Rye

- Spelt

- Sorghum

- Brown rice

- Wheat (whole or refined)

Beans - Mucus Forming:

- Black beans

- Black-eyed peas

- Bean pastas

- Broad beans

- Butter beans

- Cannellini beans

- Chickpeas (including hummus)

- Edamame

- Great Northern beans

- Italian beans

- Kidney beans

- Lentils

- Lima beans

- Mung beans

- Navy beans

- Pinto beans

- Soybeans

- Split peas

- String beans or green beans

- White beans

**Nuts and Seeds - Mucus Forming (Limit to Small Quantities or Winter Months) **:

- Acorns

- Almonds

- Brazil nuts

- Cashews

- Chestnuts

- Coconut

- Hazelnuts

- Peanuts

- Pecans

- Pistachios

- Tree nuts

- Walnuts

Processed Foods - Pus and/or Mucus Forming (Avoid):

- Convenience foods (all)

- Fast foods (all fast-food restaurants)

- Frozen convenience foods

- Packaged convenience foods

- Processed meats of all kinds

Processed Candies & Sweets - Pus and/or Highly Mucus Forming:

- Baked goods (pies, pastries, cakes, muffins, etc.)

- Candy bars

- Caramels

- Chocolate (vegan/dairy)

- Fudge

- Gelatin (Jello, gummies, etc.)

- Ice cream (dairy & non-dairy)

- Jelly candies

- Marshmallows

- Rock candy

- All candy

- Taffy

Fermented Foods - Acid Forming Stimulants:

- Ale

- Apple cider vinegar

- Barley malt syrup

- Beer

- Brandy

- Brown rice syrup

- Champagne

- Chocolate

- Chocolate syrup

- Ciders

- Cocoa

- Coffee

- Corn syrup

- Flavored syrup

- Gin

- Herbal wine

- Kombucha tea or drink

- Lager

- Liqueur

- Mead

- Port

- Rum

- Sake

- Soft drinks / Soda

- Tea

- Tequila

- Vodka

- Whiskey

- White vinegar

- Rice vinegar

- Wine

- Sherry

- White wine

Vegetarian & Vegan Processed Foods - Moderately to Highly Mucus Forming & Acid Forming:

- Chips (corn, potato, plantain, etc.)

- Frozen vegan breakfast foods (waffles, etc.)

- Hummus

- Lab-grown animal tissue

- Nutritional yeast

- Egg-free pastas

- Pasteurized fruit juices (potentially acid-forming)

- Plant milk (nut milk, seed milk, grain milk, soy milk, etc.)

- Plant-based creamers

- Plant-based yogurts

- Soy lecithin (food preservative/additive)

- Tempeh

- Texturized vegetable protein (fake/mock meats)

- Tofu

- Vegan baked goods

- Vegan breakfast cereals

- Vegan candy

- Vegan cheese substitutes

- Vegan chocolates

- Vegan ice cream

- Vegan mayonnaise

- Vegan whipped cream

Oils - Fatty and Mildly to Moderately Mucus Forming:
- Chia seed

- Citrus oil

- Coconut oil

- Corn oil

- Cottonseed oil

- Flax seed oil

- Grape seed oil

- Hemp seed oil

- Nut oils

- Olive oil

-Palm oil

- Peanut oil

- Quinoa oil

- Rapeseed (canola oil is rapeseed oil)

- Safflower oil

- Soybean oil

Salts and Spices - Stimulants and Potentially Acid-Forming:

- Black peppercorns

- Cayenne pepper

- Celery salt

- Chili powder

- Iodized salt

- Nutmeg

- Paprika

- Pepper

- Sea salt

- Vanilla extract

Please note that this information is provided as a guideline and that individual dietary choices may vary based on personal preferences and health considerations. Always consult with a qualified healthcare professional before making significant changes to your diet.

In summary, it's eye-opening to realize that a large portion of the foods we commonly consume isn't out of necessity but rather learned habits. These habits and traditions often don't support optimal health or the body's natural healing processes. While some individuals have lived long lives with meat, dairy, and eggs in their diets, closer inspection reveals limited consumption and other lifestyle factors influencing longevity. Our species' modern health challenges stem from excessive and misguided consumption, emphasizing the need to realign our choices with our well-being.

Professor Spira generously agreeing to contribute to this chapter, has provided the following passage. His expertise and willingness to share his insights have been invaluable in adding depth to this section.

Embracing Transition: The Unsung Hero of Healing

Greetings Brothers and Sisters,

Have you ever tried to change the course of a river in a single day? Or witnessed a caterpillar morph into a butterfly overnight? Nature, in her infinite wisdom, teaches us the art of patience, the beauty of progression, and the essence of transition. It is in this spirit that we delve into the often overlooked and misunderstood, yet fundamentally crucial, element of Prof. Arnold Ehret's *Mucusless Diet Healing System* – the Transition Diet.

"Everything is perfectly performed by Nature through evolutional, progressive changes," Arnold Ehret wisely observes. The Transition Diet isn't just a bridge between the unhealthy habits of the past and the vibrant, mucus-free future; it is a journey, an awakening, and a gentle harmonizing with the rhythms of our own nature.

The Transition Diet, dear reader, is not a mere footnote in the annals of natural healing; but the symphony of life that orchestrates our return to vitality! It is the gentle whisper of the wind guiding the leaves to the ground, a dance of release and renewal.

The Misunderstood Art Form

Is it not perplexing how the brilliance of the Transition Diet is often relegated to the shadows? People are eager for transformation, but the allure of instant gratification casts a veil over the profound wisdom of gradual change. "Nature's mills grind slow but sure," Ehret reminds us, yet we find ourselves racing, rushing, craving the quick fix.

Many well-meaning health-seekers perpetually fall victim to the belief that they can leap into a mucus-free, 100% raw, and/or fruit-based existence without embracing the journey of transition. It's akin to expecting a seed to sprout into a blossoming tree overnight! The Transition Diet is not a mere pitstop; it's the scenic route unveiling the landscapes of our inner ecology.

Ehret clearly emphasizes that one should adhere to "only a SLIGHT CHANGE toward an improved diet" initially. This concept, although woven intricately throughout the *Mucusless Diet* book, often eludes many who, in their pursuit to practice the diet without proficient guidance, overlook the essence of transition and leap hastily into extended periods of fasting and strict fruit dieting. The magnitude of the misstep in adopting such an approach cannot be stressed enough. Ehret explicitly dissuades any patient from embracing long fasts or protracted fruit dieting at the onset.

To put the art of the Transition Diet into perspective, consider that Ehret does not recommend the use of raw fruits for the entire first month of the transition. Instead, stewed and/or baked fruit are encouraged for fruit courses or meals, while mucus-free salads and baked vegetables round out the other meal(s). Why? Because cooked fruit is much less aggressive than raw fruit. And for someone with pounds of uneliminated feces, fecal stones, mucoid plaque, and uneliminated poisonous drugs in their system, cooked fruit proves to be a gentle eliminator, that prepares the body for the raw cleansing fruit to come.

As Ehret so eloquently put it:

> *"Everything is perfectly performed by Nature through evolutional, progressive changes, developments, and accomplishments and not by catastrophes. Nothing is more incorrect than the mistaken idea that a decades-old chronic disease can be healed through a very long fast, or a radically extended, strict fruit diet. 'Nature's mills grind slow but sure (Arnold Ehret, "Transition Diet: Lesson XV," Mucusless Diet Healing System)"*

Transition itself is not a choice. It is NATURAL LAW! Thus, our primary occupation as Earthlings is to learn how to best align ourselves with Nature.

Nature = Transition

I advocate for a reimagined perspective on transition and the transition diet. Not viewing it as an elective aspect to dabble with, but recognizing it as the quintessence of life itself.

The journey from infancy to adulthood, encompassing body and mind, is devoid of meaning without transition. Acquiring new knowledge is unattainable without transition. What we label as "seasons" in various corners of our globe are merely manifestations of Nature in transition. Fruit doesn't materialize on trees by magic, but is the culmination of transitional growth.

Transition/transformation is inescapable, and we have the choice either to resist it, deceive ourselves with the notion that we can dominate or regulate it, or to comprehend how to harmonize and align with it. It is my proposition that we embrace the latter.

Patience, dear friends, is not just a virtue; it is the art of life, a melody that harmonizes with the rhythm of our being. The Transition Diet is the canvas upon which we patiently paint our journey to wellness, with each brushstroke reflecting our commitment to gradual, mindful change.

Navigating the Culinary Landscape

Navigating the culinary landscape of the Transition Diet can be an adventure of discovery and delight! Contrary to what many people think, the Mucusless Diet is not a hymn sung only in the key of *raw foods* or a melody played solely on the *strings of fruits*. It is a grand symphony, a harmonious blend of both raw and cooked foods, a dance of variety that brings forth the song of elimination.

Ehret's wisdom guides us through the culinary journey: "The speed of elimination depends upon quantities and qualities of food and can therefore be controlled and regulated according to the condition of the patient."

An understanding of the concept of "elimination" is key. Elimination, from a Mucusless Diet perspective, may be defined as the removal of physiological wastes and encumbrances. In parlance, the term is also used instead of the word "sick" by Mucusless Diet practitioners to identify short or extended periods of intensive waste removal.

Our bodies are constantly eliminating waste. With every breath we take, we're eliminating. And when you eat mucus-free, cleansing foods, these foods aid the body in its pursuit to perfectly eliminate what the body cannot use. Yet, when the body is not eliminating properly, all manner of illnesses and suffering is the inevitable outcome.

So, what does this culinary tapestry include, you may wonder? Let's explore just a taste of the possibilities!

Cooked Delights:

Baked fruits, like apples, bananas, peaches, cherries, pears, blueberries, etc.

Lightly steamed or stewed vegetables such as kale, collard greens, broccoli, zucchini, and carrots, gently cooked to enhance their eliminative abilities.

Baked sweet potatoes, a comforting embrace of earthy sweetness and eliminative goodness.

Baked squashes, like acorn, butternut, and spaghetti, that when combined with a raw combination salad, make a perfect transitional meal.

Raw Radiance:

Leafy greens like spinach, kale, red- & green-leaf lettuce, and arugula, are a chlorophyll-rich ensemble of vitality and freshness.

Fruits, berries, and melons are the jewels of nature, bursting with flavor, vibrancy, and cleansing power.

It is strongly advised to check out the "Transition Diet" lessons of the *Mucusless Diet Healing System* to gain a full understanding of the endless possibilities of Ehret's transitional methodology.

Debunking the Raw Myth

The allure of raw foods is undeniable – the vibrancy, the freshness, the unadulterated essence of nature. It was our human ancestor's way of life. But, at some point, we humans lost our way. Thus, we must pay reparations for generations of wrong eating to transform our bodies back to the Edenic ideal. The belief that the *Mucusless Diet Healing System* is exclusively a raw or fruit-only affair is a grievous misunderstanding. The Transition Diet is a harmonious blend, a balanced composition of both raw and cooked, a celebration of diversity. When combined properly, the body will function and transform in ways that many who attempt to skip the transitional methods will never understand.

Ehret illuminated the path of balance: "A carefully selected and progressively changing TRANSITION DIET is the best and surest way for every patient to start a cure." It's not about extremes; it's about harmony. It's not about restriction; it's about exploration. It is a journey of discovery, a celebration of the myriad flavors, textures, and vital substances that nature bestows upon us. It's about tuning into our bodies, listening to its wisdom, and nourishing them with love and sacred breath. The Transition Diet invites us to groove to the rhythm of balance, to embrace the variety of nature's bounty, and to celebrate the culinary diversity that cleanses our body, mind, and spirit.

Embracing the Journey

The Transition Diet is not a detour; it's the main road, a journey marked by self-discovery, awakening, and transformation. It's about embracing the ebb and flow, the symphony of change, and the dance of life. The Transition Diet is the unsung hero of healing, the maestro orchestrating our return to harmony.

Therefore, let us celebrate the wisdom of transition, honor the journey, and dance to the melody of healing. Let us embrace the art of patience, the beauty of progression, and the essence of our true nature. The Transition Diet is our companion, our guide, and our teacher on this wondrous journey to vibrant health and mucus-free living.

In the words of the venerable Arnold Ehret, "Eat your way into Paradise physically. But you cannot pass the gate, watched over by the angel with the flaming sword, until you have gone through purgatory (cleansing fire) of fasting and diet of healing—a cleansing, a physiological purifying, by the 'Flame of Life' in your own body!"

Let us embrace Nature's powerful purification through a transitional "diet of healing" toward a Mucus-free Life with open hearts, open minds, and a renewed spirit, for it is the gateway to our Physiological Liberation!

Peace, Love, and Breath!

Prof. Spira
September 2023
mucusfreelife.com

Chapter 11
Comparing Different Approaches

Now that I've shared dietary advice from Arnold Ehret, Dr. Joel Fuhrman, Dr. John McDougall, and Natural Hygiene, it's interesting to look at how their dietary and lifestyle recommendations compare. There are notable similarities and significant differences that warrant discussion. Reflecting on the sequence in which I learned and shared this information, it almost felt like a progression from less strict to more disciplined approaches. I believe that if I had encountered these insights in a different order, my understanding and level of health wouldn't be as fortunate as they are today.

My journey into health and the importance of adopting a plant-based diet for healing began with the book «The PH Miracle» by Dr. Robert O. Young. His guidance helped me transition from my previous organic farm diet (including meat, raw dairy, eggs, etc.) to a health-promoting «Mucusless Plant Diet.» A few months later, I came across Arnold Ehret's teachings from the early 1900s, after incorporating Dr. Young's dietary principles into my routine. Dr. Robert Young's recommendations included grains and fish (the only animal-based food), which I included in my diet for a short time before fully embracing Arnold Ehret's 100% plant-based approach. Looking back, Dr. Young's teachings acted as a necessary steppingstone that allowed me to grasp and understand Arnold Ehret's timeless wisdom without finding it too extreme. Without Dr. Young's initial guidance, I'm uncertain if I would have comprehended Ehret's teachings to the same extent.

Over the years, I've received feedback from people who attempted to read Arnold Ehret's writings based on my recommendations. It appears that some either misinterpret his message or struggle to comprehend his teachings. It's possible that Ehret's language, being from a different time (about 100 years ago), contributes to this challenge, or there might be other unknown factors. Our current mindset and beliefs strongly influence how we interpret information, and our existing health status could also play a role in the misinterpretation of his work. This is one of the motivations behind writing this book. By initially incorporating Dr. Young›s insights in the early stages of my journey, I was better equipped to understand the health-preserving knowledge that Arnold Ehret offered. As the saying goes, «When the student is ready, the teacher appears."

Personal Evolution in Perspective

 My perspective on consuming meat has undergone a significant transformation over the past 11 years. Back when I lived on a farm, witnessing the killing and processing of animals, I deemed it an extreme practice on multiple fronts. The cruelty, messiness, labor-intensive nature, and the entire process involved in bringing meat to the table struck me as a profoundly intricate endeavor. It›s intriguing how people may not be willing to undertake this process themselves, yet they consume store-bought meat with little thought about the behind-the-scenes efforts. It›s worth mentioning that government subsidies play a substantial role in keeping meat and dairy affordable; without them, fewer people might opt for these items. The effort and cost associated with bringing these products to market far surpass what the price tags suggest, but government policies appear to encourage consumption. This underlines how mindset and external factors shape our dietary choices.

Reflecting on my mindset, I recall watching the documentary "Forks Over Knives" during my farm days. Back then, I found the documentary extreme and almost amusing in its approach. However, upon rewatching it years later, after embracing a plant-based diet, the documentary resonated deeply, and its message felt entirely different. This shift in perspective exemplifies how our level of health profoundly influences our understanding and interpretation of information. It's clear that our internal toxicity can greatly affect how we perceive external influences.

My journey towards better health followed a serendipitous

path. After gradually eliminating mucus-forming, disease-promoting foods from my diet and living as mucus-free as possible for about two years, I came across Dr. Robert Morse's teachings. His insights coincided with my aspiration to enhance my diet. Inspired by Dr. Morse's guidance, I transitioned towards consuming predominantly fruits and raw foods for the next year. During this phase, I experienced various episodes of elimination and healing. One instance involved a swollen jaw that rendered eating painful for over a week. Inevitably, my food intake decreased, and I unintentionally fasted for a few days. As my body coped with this challenge, I experienced delirious fever-like night sweats for about 24 hours. The pain was excruciating, even pushing me to contemplate hospitals or pain medication, which was uncharacteristic of me. Yet, I persisted, refraining from intervening with my body's natural healing process. Miraculously, the fever subsided, my jaw healed, and I emerged from this experience strengthened. It became evident that oftentimes, doing "nothing intelligently" is the most intelligent course of action in aiding the body's innate healing mechanisms.

Advancing Through New Insights

Continuing the journey, a year or two later, fresh perspectives emerged—this time, through the teachings of Natural Hygiene. These teachings steered me towards a more holistic approach to refining my dietary and lifestyle practices, beyond the exclusive focus on fruits with minimal greens. Integrating Natural Hygiene principles aligned and harmonized much of what I had gleaned from Dr. Morse, Arnold Ehret, and other sources. However, it also prompted me to discern some less optimal recommendations offered by Dr. Robert Morse.

The teachings on herbs presented by Natural Hygiene took me by surprise, yet the timing was perfect. By this point, my own experiences in supporting others› healing journeys through herbal supplements and tinctures had equipped me to appreciate the truths being presented. Interestingly, my personal observations had already hinted at the negative effects of herbs, despite their supposed medicinal attributes. People I worked with often reported a sense of imbalance and slower healing, contrary to the anticipated benefits. Natural Hygiene provided the insights that resonated with my growing suspicions, elucidating the underlying reasons for these observations. During this period, I was actively engaged in health consultations, assisting others on their paths to wellness.

It›s almost surreal to acknowledge that years invested in the study of «Herbal Medicine,» delving into the purported healing properties of various herbs, could be based on misconceptions and incomplete truths. The frustration stems from realizing that a substantial portion of the knowledge disseminated on herbal remedies may be inaccurate, and more alarmingly, potentially harmful to human well-being. The global consensus around herbal «medicine» perpetuates a narrative that has been upheld for centuries. Challenging this consensus can seem ludicrous, considering the weight of history and tradition.

A couple more years down the line, while still adhering to a high-raw, high-fruit diet, I reached a point where I could finally proclaim freedom from lingering health symptoms. I had dedicated years to enhancing my dietary and lifestyle choices, gradually attaining levels of health previously uncharted in my experience. The healing process wasn›t without challenges, as overcoming my extensive list of health issues demanded commitment and effort. Although I successfully vanquished most symptoms, occasional headaches persisted. The revelation of the root cause of these headaches, as shared in the «Headaches» chapter, shed light on a crucial aspect that had eluded teachings from Dr. Morse, Arnold Ehret, and others—the significance of water. Sometimes, answers lie in seemingly minor details that, when incorporated, yield transformative outcomes. Often, it's the subtle elements that evade our attention, yet possess the potency to revolutionize our well-being. In essence, simplicity holds profound power.

A Journey of Exploration and Insight

My fascination with health has grown into a passion over the past decade, propelling me to continually study and delve into the topic. Just last year, I immersed myself in the teachings of modern plant-based doctors like Dr. John McDougall and Dr. Joel Fuhrman, absorbing their distinct dietary approaches—the Starch Solution for Dr. McDougall and the G-Bombs approach for Dr. Fuhrman. This thirst for knowledge led me to undertake a self-experiment with the Starch Solution diet, not only to uncover the truth about starch but also to speak about it from personal experience. Numerous inquiries from people over the years about Dr. McDougall›s dietary protocol had spurred me to explore this firsthand.

It›s intriguing how feeling good health-wise can sometimes lead to losing sight of essential truths and veering off track. The memory of living in pain might recede into the distant past, almost as if it never occurred. While I don›t regret the 75-day experiment with the Starch Solution diet—even though it took a toll on my health—it ultimately reinforced my understanding of starch›s impact on the body. This experience was pivotal in clarifying the truth, dispelling any doubts.

If I were to embark on another dietary experiment, I›d consider Dr. Joel Fuhrman›s recommendations. His guidance offers reasonable dietary advice, and his approach is less commonly perceived as extreme compared to some other perspectives like Arnold Ehret, Dr. Morse, and Natural Hygiene. Dr. Fuhrman›s insights might be suitable for transitioning away from harmful foods, although some of his specific recommendations, like consuming raw onions daily or regularly including beans, raise questions for me. Incorporating beans with ample leafy greens to aid digestion and elimination seems a more balanced approach. Despite my reservations, I recognize the value of his guidance for those seeking a pragmatic transition.

Reflecting on my Starch Solution experiment, I realize that my deep familiarity with the «Mucusless Diet Healing System» for several years prior prompted my curiosity. The experiment sought to assess the impact of reintroducing starches into my diet after a long period of absence. Despite having excluded starches from my diet for years following my embrace of Arnold Ehret›s teachings, this experiment offered insights into their effects when reintroduced within a healthy plant-based context. However, several variables influenced the outcomes.

I want to clarify that a diet like the Starch Solution, when adjusted to include a lesser proportion of starches (as opposed to the recommended 90%), could be a sound starting point for individuals seeking a healthier path, especially if they aren't purists. Such a protocol helps relieve health issues and initiates a process of eliminating burdensome dietary elements. True health often hinges on elimination, removing irritating, stimulating, and disease-promoting foods. Dr. Fuhrman's or Dr. McDougall's dietary frameworks naturally induce the removal of unnatural foods that likely contributed to initial symptoms.

 Interestingly, during my Starch Solution trial, I noticed that my meal sizes were excessive, especially at dinner. Over time, my commitment to a 100% raw food diet has highlighted that cooked food tends to lead to overeating—this seems to hold true for myself and many others. This insight aligns with Dr. Joel Fuhrman›s teachings about the harmful effects of overeating. Reflecting on my Starch Solution experience, it›s evident that the manner of consumption played a role in the overall impact on my health.

 Although hitting «rock bottom» during my Starch Solution experiment was challenging, it served as a stark reminder of the pain I once endured. This painful episode reaffirmed the unyielding determination to avoid returning to a life of suffering. It solidified truths I had already known, and I adjusted my eating habits accordingly to ensure freedom from headaches. In hindsight, this experience was a powerful catalyst for realigning with health and recommitting to a pain-free existence.

Adapting Recommendations to Meet Individuals Where They Are

To truly help others, we must tailor our advice to their unique situations. For instance, it wouldn›t be practical to suggest that a meat eater unfamiliar with Natural Hygienic principles suddenly switch to a diet of just fruits, greens, and minimal plant fats for optimal health. Transitioning away from addictive foods is a gradual process. Our recommendations should align with their readiness, goals, and willingness to make changes.

It›s essential to consider what works for them, not impose the ideal immediately, as everyone's journey is distinct. To guide effectively, we must understand their health priorities, sacrifices, and aspirations. For those transitioning from Standard Diets rich in meats, the Starch Solution Diet could be a suitable starting point. Someone on a vegetarian diet seeking improvement might benefit from Dr. Joel Fuhrman's approach. It's about meeting them where they are, rather than where we are.

My perspective on the Starch Solution Diet is that it›s a healthy introduction to plant-based eating. It can serve as a long-term option for those who desire a healthier plant-based or vegan diet without complete transformation. Dr. Fuhrman›s recommendations could be a progressive step after the Starch Solution Diet, offering improvement. Even if someone simply reduces meat consumption based on the information shared, it›s a positive outcome.

For those pursuing utmost health and willing to embrace more drastic changes, referring them to older publications from the 1700s to the 1900s can provide valuable insights. The plant-based vegan path offers a spectrum of disciplines, allowing individuals to choose their level of commitment, typically leading to positive results.

From my personal experience, a high raw/fruit diet supplemented with some cooked vegetables during dinner has shown me the optimal nature of a raw food diet for humans.

However, a gradual transition is crucial, especially if shifting from a previous diet. A raw food diet is more manageable in warmer climates with access to fresh, ripe fruit year-round, but proper transition is vital. For a deeper understanding of the importance of the transition diet, Arnold Ehret›s books «The Mucusless Diet Healing System» and «Rational Fasting» offer in-depth insights.

If Arnold Ehret were alive today, he might be shocked by the existence of the "SSD" diet. The differences between the two approaches are striking. The "Mucusless Diet Healing System" emphasizes avoiding all starches as they are considered "Mucus Forming Foods" for the human body. Instead, it suggests consuming fruits, leafy greens, and cooked starchless vegetables. On the other hand, the SSD promotes starches as the healthiest foods, with only small amounts of fruits, greens, and starchless vegetables included.

After my 75-day trial with the SSD, I returned to my healing dietary routine of raw fruits, vegetables, and leafy greens. These foods helped me overcome a range of health issues. Transitioning to a 100% raw food diet took time, as I gradually eliminated steamed and cooked vegetables. I allowed my body to guide me, eventually making the switch when it felt right and effortless.

Incorporating Natural Hygienic principles elevated my health to the next level. While my SSD experiment brought unnecessary challenges, it taught me valuable lessons. The Mucusless Diet Healing System remains my foundation, where even steamed and baked vegetables became my «junk food» or «cheat» treats—a sign of progress.

This lifestyle isn›t a rigid «diet» but a mindful integration of knowledge about foods that benefit our species. I›ve shaped my eating habits to include one or two fruit meals earlier in the day and a substantial raw, leafy green salad with raw veggies, fruits, and homemade dressing for dinner. Things fell into place naturally when I allowed rather than forced the process.

Eliminating disease-causing foods and healing my once deemed «incurable» health problems ranks among my top three achievements. Discovering this life-changing information, even in a world resistant to change, has been profoundly rewarding. I overcame skepticism and mockery to achieve a remarkable level of health. Since April 2023 marks nine years since I learned about a meat and dairy-free option, I›m reminded of my journey. Back then, I wasn›t aware of the possibility, and my suffering stemmed from conventional dietary beliefs.

Are Plant-Based Fats Beneficial for Health?

Arnold Ehret held the belief that fats, including plant-based fats, were not conducive to human health. He discouraged the consumption of avocados, nuts, seeds, fatty fruits, and processed oils as they were deemed mucus-forming, constipating, and digestion-slowing. Ehret suggested limited consumption of nuts and seeds during winter.

Dr. Robert Morse's perspective allows for avocado, fatty fruits, and coconut in a regular raw food diet, yet he cautions against daily consumption of plant fats during detoxification or healing. He highlights their potential to impede detoxification and recommends soaking or sprouting nuts and seeds before consuming them in small amounts due to their protein and phytic acid content.

Dr. John McDougall's stance emphasizes that "the fat we eat is the fat we wear". He asserts that fats, particularly processed oils, lack health benefits in the human diet. While he permits modest intake of seeds or avocado for those not seeking weight loss, he associates fat consumption with weight gain.

Natural Hygiene supports the inclusion of whole, raw plant fats—like Nuts, Seeds, Avocado, and Coconut—in moderation (within 5-10% of daily intake) for a healthy diet. Processed fats in the form of refined oils are discouraged, in line with Natural Hygiene's belief that processed foods burden the body.

Dr. Joel Fuhrman advises limited fat intake, suggesting no more than 2 ounces of avocado, or an ounce of nuts per day, and a tablespoon of ground flax seeds (or hemp seeds) daily. This aligns with his emphasis on minimal fat consumption for health.

My Thoughts on Fats: Limiting Nuts and Seeds for Health

I believe that consuming excessive nuts and seeds isn't health-promoting (and they're quite easy to overeat). I share Arnold Ehret's view (and Natural Hygiene) that nuts and seeds should be consumed moderately and primarily during the winter months. This aligns with their role as preserved, complex foods that are available when fresh options are scarce.

When I transitioned to a 100% raw diet, I started using Nuts and Seeds in my diet as creamy salad dressings rather than eating them whole. I blend nuts or seeds (usually sunflower or hemp seeds) with vegetables for these dressings. This approach prevents daily fat overload, which is a potential issue if I were to consume them whole.

I've noticed that the raw food community often relies on plant fats like avocados, nuts, seeds, and fatty fruits for satiety. Many raw food dishes in restaurants and on social media contain substantial amounts of these fats, often labeled as «gourmet raw foods.» While I've tried these dishes, I've found that the high protein content in nuts can leave me with a slight food hangover due to my body's lack of familiarity with regular nut consumption.

I think having half an avocado with a salad is acceptable occasionally for satiety, despite its somewhat mucus-forming and constipating properties. Pairing it with a leafy green salad aids digestion, absorption, and movement. Feeling satisfied helps curb less healthy cravings. Fats are best consumed with greens and not combined with sugars, even fruits—proper food combining is vital.

From my personal experience and research, I believe that the recommendation of minimal nuts, seeds, and plant fats is widely agreed upon. Personally, I feel my best when I consume these fats sparingly. Overdoing fats can negatively impact health; our bodies aren›t designed for high fat intake. In Nature, the effort required to forage and crack nuts balances their consumption. We tend to overeat nuts and seeds now that they›re conveniently available in stores.

Healthy fats are only beneficial when not overconsumed. Excess fat can hinder nutrient absorption and create a coating on intestinal walls, leading to malabsorption issues overtime often mistaken for nutrient deficiencies. Prolonged excessive fat intake is risky. Ideally, overt fats should not be a daily staple. For instance, an average person weighing 150 pounds shouldn't exceed half an avocado or a handful of nuts or seeds per day. Raw food desserts often contain excessive nuts and seeds, making them easy to overindulge in.

Are Supplements and Herbs Beneficial for Health?

Arnold Ehret, to the best of my knowledge, didn't advocate for them much, except for occasional use of mild laxative herbs in extreme cases.

Dr. Robert Morse is a strong proponent of herbal support. He's developed an extensive range of herbal products, including tinctures, loose tea blends, and capsules. Dr. Morse asserts that substances other than herbs, like supplements and isolates, may burden the body and contribute to toxicity. He believes that only whole foods, like herbs, are fully recognized and utilized by the body, promoting healing.

Dr. John McDougall takes a different stance, surprising for a medical doctor. He doesn't endorse supplements, claiming that a well-balanced diet can supply all necessary nutrients. Although he acknowledges using a B12 supplement, he does so mainly as a precaution and for legal reasons.

According to **Natural Hygiene**, true health stems from a diet of whole plant foods. NH asserts that the body can self-heal without external substances. While herbs are said to act on the body, Natural Hygiene emphasizes the body's role in interacting with herbs, cautioning against their use and the use of other all substances.

Dr. Joel Fuhrman recommends the inclusion of vitamins and supplements. He believes deficiencies increase chronic disease risks and offers supplements on his website, with a focus on Vitamin D, B12, and vitamins K1 and K2.

My Thoughts on Supplements

I'm grateful that I've used very few herbs or substances throughout my life. In the past 9+ years, the only time I ventured into herbs was when I followed Dr. Morse's guidance. I gave some of his tinctures a try but quickly abandoned them, realizing they weren't right for me. Avoiding supplements and substances has spared me from confusion and misinterpretation that often surrounds them. Those who dive into the world of vitamins and herbs often struggle to discern what's true.

I›ve never relied on «protein powders,» vitamins, or supplements, which I consider fortunate as it spared my body from unnecessary burden. Before embracing a plant-based vegan diet, I experimented with harmful substances like Diatomaceous Earth and Colloidal Silver. Thankfully, I realized their limited benefits and stopped using them. I›m fortunate that I didn›t get into supplements or vitamins, even during pregnancy when Folic Acid was recommended. Instinctively, I couldn›t bring myself to take it.

I fully agree with Natural Hygiene›s teachings that vitamins, supplements, powders, herbs, and substances offer no benefit. The body thrives on whole, natural foods, and these substances only burden it, building toxicity. Dr. Morse shares this perspective, aligning with Natural Hygiene except for herbal medicine.

At best, the body eliminates supplements and such as waste. Contrary to popular belief, substances don›t act on the body; the body acts on them. The body›s efforts to rid itself of harmful substances are often misinterpreted as beneficial effects. Working with many individuals, I›ve witnessed how simplifying their approach by eliminating supplements and herbs leads to significant health improvements.

It›s unusual in today›s world not to reach for something when symptoms arise. However, symptoms are the body›s way of trying to heal itself. Suppressing them with substances can harm our health. Taking absolutely nothing might feel strange to many, but investing in whole, natural foods is the true path to healthcare.

Vinegars

Arnold Ehret and **Dr. Robert Morse** advise against consuming vinegars or fermented foods, as they believe these contribute to acidity within the body and can worsen fungal issues.

Dr. John McDougall approves of vinegar consumption within certain limits. He permits vinegars in processed condiments like ketchup and salad dressings, provided they are free from salt, oil, and sugar. He focuses on starch consumption but doesn't emphasize the acidic nature of these condiments.

Natural Hygiene discourages vinegar consumption due to its processed nature and acid-forming properties. Vinegar is not a whole food in its natural state and is considered burdensome for the body.

Dr. Joel Fuhrman, on the other hand, supports vinegar consumption and offers flavored vinegar products for sale on his website.

My Thoughts on Vinegars

I wish vinegars were good for health, but I'm not a fan of using them regularly, even though I can tolerate a bit of balsamic or apple cider vinegar in dressings or sauces (though I don't use them myself). Vinegar can harm tooth enamel if consumed frequently. I've only knowingly had vinegar a handful of times over the past 9+ years. I find white vinegar too strong, although I use it for housecleaning. Balsamic and apple cider vinegar are more acceptable to me, yet I prefer using lemon as a "Healthy Food Swap." I agree with Arnold Ehret, Natural Hygiene, and Dr. Robert Morse that vinegars aren't beneficial for health. They're highly acidic, burden the body, and can harm teeth and overall health over time. I once heard a podcast by the Medical Medium explaining why vinegars are unhealthy, and it made sense. If someone does consume vinegar, the least harmful option might be Apple Cider Vinegar, though it's still not an ideal choice. I used Apple Cider Vinegar to remove a skin tag from my neck in the past. It burned off the skin tag in about 5 days, but I had to wait for the redness and inflammation to heal afterward. It's quite remarkable how powerful vinegar can be – if it can dissolve a skin tag in such a short time, I wonder about its effects inside our bodies. Regular vinegar consumption seems risky, almost like playing with fire. When I think of vinegar, I picture inflammation in a bottle.

Is Juicing Fresh Fruits / Vegetables Healthy?

Arnold Ehret believed in the benefits of fresh juices as they are "mucusless" and aid in hydrating the body and removing old waste. He considered fresh juice mucusless and thus acceptable.

Dr. Robert Morse supports fruit juicing for detoxification and healing purposes. He suggests fruit juice cleanses for deep healing while maintaining daily activities. According to Dr. Morse, fruit juices provide hydration, cleansing, and health benefits without burdening digestion.

Dr. John McDougall cautioned against juicing, stating it separates whole foods into less beneficial parts. He emphasized a starch-based diet for optimal health and did not endorse juicing.

Natural Hygiene discourages juicing, as it removes fiber and processes foods unnaturally. Chewing whole foods is vital for proper assimilation, digestion, and dental health, which juicing compromises.

Dr. Joel Fuhrman recommends green juices as part of a "Nutritarian" diet, with a caution against excessive fruit due to calorie density, favoring more vegetables.

My Thoughts on Juicing

I've juiced fruits quite a bit over the years. Personally, I never juiced vegetables or greens because I don't enjoy their taste, and I don't eat anything my body rejects. If something doesn't taste good, it's a sign not to consume it. However, some people dislike healthy foods due to being accustomed to unhealthy diets, so this isn't always true.

A few years back, I tried juicing celery for its reported health benefits, but I found the taste unappealing and stopped. I've done 14-day fruit juice cleanses before, but that was before I learned about Natural Hygiene. Juicing can be a helpful transition tool, but it shouldn't replace whole meals. Chewing is crucial for dental health, which juicing can affect.

Juicing can improve hydration for chronically dehydrated individuals and aid in transitioning from unhealthy beverages. However, it should not replace daily salads or whole fruit meals. Extended juice cleanses can lead to dental and health issues. Juicing is a tool, not a long-term solution.

While juicing helped me transition, I believe in focusing on healthy dietary habits and using juicing occasionally. It doesn't replace a healthy diet. People often benefit from juicing due to eliminating unhealthy foods. I juice only to use excess fruit and keep the pulp for digestion. I've avoided teeth issues over the years by balancing fruit with daily greens and chewing my food.

Ultimately, I've realized that eating whole fruits is more natural and satisfying than juice. Juicing can be beneficial in moderation, but it's not necessary for building health. It's essential to focus on a balanced, healthy diet and use juicing as a temporary aid.

Enemas, a method of cleaning the lower intestines – Yes, or No?

Arnold Ehret advocates daily enemas to remove accumulated waste and toxins. He views enemas as internal showers, aiding in purifying the body and eliminating impurities. Ehret suggests regular enemas until the body is free of waste.

Dr. Robert Morse prefers herbal methods to stimulate bowel movement instead of enemas. He believes herbs assist the body in eliminating toxins rather than acting on the body directly.

Dr. John McDougall's stance on enemas is unclear, as he hasn't addressed the topic in his work to my knowledge. Given his medical background, he might discourage at-home procedures and emphasize dietary changes.

Natural Hygiene rejects enemas, stating that the body naturally controls elimination and that enema's are enervating. Forcing the process weakens the body, and the digestive tract is meant for exit only. Natural Hygiene advocates a return to natural dietary and lifestyle practices for self-cleansing.

Dr. Joel Fuhrman supports enemas, including coffee enemas, as a means of detoxification. His website features articles promoting various enema methods, such as those with Epsom salts, probiotics, and colostrum.

My Thoughts on Enemas

I used to believe enemas were beneficial and followed Arnold Ehret's advice. During my initial years of pursuing health, I did enemas. However, as I gained more knowledge, my perspective changed. Now, I agree with Natural Hygiene, which asserts that enemas weaken colon muscles and can be enervating. Hospitals once used enemas to address health issues caused by backed-up waste, but this medical treatment comes with its own costs.

In my early healing journey, I didn't notice the negative effects described by Natural Hygiene. Yet, this doesn't guarantee no harm was done, as we can't see everything inside our bodies. At times, I felt weak due to detoxification, which diverts nerve energy from muscles. I eventually stopped enemas, except for during headaches, before realizing water intake and healthier living were better solutions.

Enemas not only weaken but can stretch and detach the colon's muscle wall, posing risks. Our bodies eliminate waste naturally and should be allowed to do so on their schedule. If there's a problem, improving dietary and lifestyle habits is the way to go. After numerous enemas, I now see their harm and unnaturalness. Recommending or using enemas isn't part of a healthful equation; building healthy habits is the key to true well-being.

Is Salt Healthy?

- **Arnold Ehret** sees added salt as potentially stimulating and acid-forming within the body.

- **Dr. Robert Morse** believes all salt is non-health-promoting and not suitable for a diet focused on raw foods, especially fruits.

- **Dr. John McDougall** acknowledges salt's lack of health promotion but suggests using a little for taste, post-cooking.

- **Natural Hygiene** asserts that all salts contain toxic inorganic minerals, leading to impaired metabolic functions and water retention.

- **Dr. Joel Fuhrman** links salt to health risks like high blood pressure, heart issues, and cancer, warning against its overuse.

 Overall, the consensus leans toward avoiding salt due to its potential negative effects on health.

My Thoughts on Salt

I agree that salts are harmful to health – they act like poison in the body. Salt leads to water retention and weight gain, causing dehydration and lymphatic congestion. It works as a diuretic, draining our energy and hindering our lymphatic system. Salt's inorganic nature can harm us over time, especially if adrenal health is compromised. It may stimulate temporarily but doesn't address the root cause. I cut out salt years ago, and now I neither crave nor like it. If I do have salt, I notice facial puffiness and fatigue the next day. Quitting salt wasn't easy; I substituted dehydrated ground celery to transition. Over time, my taste adapted, and my body healed. In a natural context, salt wouldn't be a regular part of our diets. Many are salt-addicted, but I believe there's no real advantage to consuming it. If a dish needs salt to taste good, the food might not be the right choice.

Is Honey Beneficial for Health?

 Opinions on honey›s healthiness vary among experts.

 Arnold Ehret argues that honey, being "Mucusless," is suitable for regular consumption due to its alignment with a Mucusless diet and proper elimination. He views honey as a "mucusless food" that supports health.

Dr. Robert Morse opposes honey as a sweetener, citing its acid-forming nature. He advocates consuming whole, natural foods without the need for sweeteners. Fruits, in his view, are delicious on their own.

Dr. John McDougall permits honey as a food addition if it helps individuals stick to his starch-based diet. He prioritizes adherence to his diet plan and believes honey can be included if it aligns with his recommendations.

Natural Hygiene sees honey as an acid-forming, antibiotic substance that impedes the body's natural healing and detoxification mechanisms, likening its effect to certain drugs. Honey is toxic and can be compared with eating white sugar containing no minerals or vitamins. Honey is essentially bee vomit.

Dr. Joel Fuhrman advises avoiding honey and sweeteners like maple syrup and sugar. He points out that excessive sweetness can lead to cravings and weight gain.

My Thoughts on Honey and Beekeeping

I have my own perspective on honey that might not align with all vegans, but I ask you to hear me out if you are one. I personally don›t use honey or any sweeteners other than dates – they sweeten things perfectly. While I can›t say for sure if Natural Hygienic teachings are accurate about honey being an antibiotic and highly acidic, I also can›t confirm if Arnold Ehret›s stance that honey is harmless due to its «mucusless» nature is correct. It›s clear that honey is a concentrated sweetener, and in nature, accessing a hive in a tree isn›t easy. That said, I›ve developed my own thoughts on this topic over time.

Back when I lived off the grid and cared for beehives, I realized that the vegan community›s stance against honey might not be entirely accurate. While many commercial beekeepers prioritize profits over the bees› well-being, some conscientious beekeepers genuinely care for their bees. From an ethical perspective, I don›t believe all honey use contributes to bee abuse.

In today›s world, bees face challenges like forest fires and habitat loss. I believe they need the support of beekeepers who care for their well-being. While I agree that taking honey from naturally occurring hives could be considered stealing, well-managed beekeeping might be a different scenario. We can›t equate this to wild animals vs. farm animals as it›s a unique situation.

Ethical beekeepers can provide a safe environment for bees that they might not find in the wild today. Beekeeping requires knowledge, time, and attention. Proper hive maintenance, including hive cleaning, helps prevent swarming and supports bee health. However, unethical beekeeping practices can be harmful.

If honey comes from an ethical beekeeper, I don›t see an issue with consuming excess honey as it supports responsible bee farming. While most commercial honeys might not be suitable for consumption, I›m unsure if honey is healthy. It might not be health-promoting, but consuming it occasionally is likely better than processed sugars or harmful sweeteners.

In nature, accessing honey would likely result in stings, suggesting it might not be meant for humans. Personally, I wouldn't recommend honey unless someone is managing hives ethically. A health-promoting diet shouldn't require added sweeteners; fruit's natural sweetness suffices. Scientific studies advocating honey's benefits often make me curious about the opposite view.

While I understand the vegan stance, my beekeeping experiences have shown me the complexities. Ethical beekeeping can help bees thrive in today›s world, but unethical practices harm their reputation. In a food system controlled by profit, it›s hard to ensure ethical practices. Beekeeping can be both beneficial and harmful to bees depending on intentions and practices.

Common Agreements Among Health Experts

In the realm of health and healing, it's rare to find one person or source with all the right answers. However, when several brilliant minds or modalities agree on certain points, it's wise to take note, considering the vast sea of conflicting information. While exceptions exist, agreement among these luminaries is noteworthy.

Arnold Ehret, Dr. Morse, Dr. John McDougall, Dr. Joel Fuhrman, and Natural Hygienic teachings all concur that animal products and meats, including fish, dairy, and eggs, aren't health-promoting. They contribute to toxicity and eventual disease in the body. I've personally experienced this and align with their perspective. Over nine years without animal products, I've seen its transformative effects on my health.

Another shared view is that processed oils (like Canola, Olive, and Coconut) are detrimental to health. These oils, pure liquid fats, are calorie-dense and not found naturally. They're widely recognized as unhealthy and can contribute to health issues, backed by studies presented by Dr. McDougall.

Similarly, Arnold Ehret, Natural Hygiene, and Dr. Morse caution against vinegars and fermented foods. While Dr. McDougall and Dr. Fuhrman permit vinegar use, all agree that excessive acid-forming foods can harm health. While vinegars occasionally used in moderation might be acceptable, they can erode tooth enamel and lead to health issues.

One point of unanimous agreement is that the optimal diet for health isn't merely a diet, but a lifestyle. A whole-food, plant-based, vegan diet is recommended by all five experts, though their approaches may differ. Dr. Morse emphasizes a detoxifying fruit-based diet for healing and a raw food diet for maintenance. Natural Hygiene suggests that a balanced diet, including leafy greens, raw whole fruits and raw veggie fruits, with minimal plant fats maintain health. Arnold Ehret advocates transitioning properly to a high fruit, raw food diet to accommodate our body's adaptation process.

Transitioning to a new diet is crucial, yet often overlooked. Rapid changes can lead to discomfort and failure. The consensus is that gradual shifts are key for success, allowing both body and mind to adapt to changes. This approach respects our lifelong routines and minimizes the stress of sudden transformations.

Dr. Morse, Ehret, and Natural Hygiene emphasize that humans are naturally frugivores, not Omnivores or Carnivores as commonly believed. Dr. McDougall's term "starchitarians" is close but misses the mark, omitting a crucial dietary element – fruit and its beneficial sugars. While Dr. Joel Fuhrman's "nutritarian" approach might lack emphasis on fruits due to his focus on nutrient-rich foods, it's worth noting that all agree on the frugivore nature of the human diet.

My Final Thoughts:

In the realm of health and diets, there's a lot of confusion. Many experts agree that a whole food vegan diet is best, but there are various interpretations within the vegan umbrella. I've personally tried different approaches: Dr. McDougall's starch-based plan, Ehret's mucusless diet, Dr. Morse's fruit-focused protocol, and now Natural Hygiene's raw food approach. From my 9+ years' experience, I've found that simple, raw fruits and greens work best for me.

Complex starches like potatoes and rice can burden digestion, but occasional consumption with ample water is okay. Ideally, we'd thrive on raw, unaltered foods without spices or additives. For health and healing, I avoid these starches and focus on fruits and greens. Eating twice a day with fruit snacks feels right, while heavy meals can be taxing.

Eating with the seasons, fasting occasionally, and not eating too early in the morning are practices I follow. Unfortunately, Western diets lead to poor health early. We can age gracefully by making informed dietary choices. Hydration is crucial; our diet should be hydrating, not dehydrating. Just like other creatures, we need a species-appropriate diet for optimal health.

I've experienced misery and health, so I know the impact of choices. Health is a choice, but occasional deviations are fine under the plant diet umbrella. Understanding our choices is key. The health movement is growing, challenging disease-forming foods. Change is gradual, just like health's progression. It's important to focus on our own health goals but to also set a positive example for others to follow. People will sometimes listen to what you have to say, but they will always WATCH what you do and how you do it.

Chapter 12
Making Healthy Food Swaps and Navigating the Transition Diet

Learning how to make healthier versions of the foods we're used to eating is the first step in moving towards a healthier diet. This helps us transition without feeling overwhelmed by all the changes we need to make. Using healthier food options also eases the load on our digestive system, which is crucial during this transition. Let me explain further.

The idea behind transitioning is to gradually make better choices in our diet. Over time, these changes lead us to our goal of a healthier, healing, and energizing way of eating. If you're aiming to improve your health or deal with specific health issues, it's important to understand why a gradual transition is beneficial. Everyone's situation is unique, and some might not have the luxury of taking things at their own pace due to their health condition. Changing from our old eating habits to a healthier diet requires motivation, especially during the first year or two. But if you stick with it and understand what's needed for your health, eventually, eating foods that benefit your body will become as natural as brushing your teeth. Our cravings can shift to foods that support our health. What we eat today influences what we'll crave tomorrow. Remember, building healthier habits takes time and patience, but it's achievable for everyone, regardless of their circumstances.

Nature is always changing, and we can learn from this. Understanding the process of transitioning to healthier dietary choices at our own pace ensures we enjoy each step and get creative with preparing more wholesome versions of the foods we crave. Embracing a health-conscious lifestyle isn't about depriving ourselves; it's about abundance. Nutrient-rich, hydrating foods can be enjoyed in larger quantities compared to the calorie-dense, fatty foods we're accustomed to. Eating healthily becomes a fresh way of life, opening new possibilities once we overcome the challenges of adopting new habits. The transition diet bridges the gap between where we are and where we want to be, avoiding extremes and roadblocks.

The reason for a gradual dietary shift lies in how it benefits our digestive system. By slowly transitioning to healthier habits, we ease the workload on our digestive system, freeing up energy for cleaning and healing. This prompts the body to periodically release stored waste acids into circulation for elimination. While this is ultimately beneficial, proceeding slowly is recommended. Speeding up this process can lead to discomfort and symptoms like itchy skin, fatigue, irritability, and rashes. Going slowly helps manage these effects. Rushing can lead to confusion and doubt, making you think the healthier diet isn't working. Learning from those who've gone through this process is important. Focusing solely on every symptom that arises during the body's cleansing can cause confusion and stress. My own understanding of this process, influenced by Arnold Ehret's work, helped me navigate through various symptoms. During my first year of changing my diet, my skin felt like it was crawling for weeks. I experienced swelling and frequent restroom visits. This was my body's way of adjusting to newfound hydration and detoxification. Frequent urination indicates toxin release due to years of dehydration from unnatural diets. It takes time to rehydrate and cleanse the body. Such symptoms are common among newcomers to our "Terrain Model Diet Support Group." Around 100 people join each month and report similar experiences.

When we make changes to detoxify our bodies and become healthier, something remarkable happens. We start to understand what our bodies truly need. This leads us to know when it's time to improve our diet even more, or when it's best to stick with where we are for a while. In today's world, we need to become our own health experts if we want to get better. Striking a balance is crucial. Extreme approaches can cause more problems and upset our body's balance. That's why learning the art of a transition diet is essential for long-term success. It helps us deal with pressures from society and family that could otherwise steer us away from our goals.

By using a transition diet and choosing healthier foods, we can progress at our own pace, avoiding sudden detox symptoms, rapid weight loss, and the mental struggle against cravings.

It's okay to take things slow. Just as we gradually developed poor health over time, we can slowly build back our health. This process is not something to rush, even though we might be eager or desperate to heal. It took time to create the internal toxicity that led to our symptoms, so it makes sense that reversing those symptoms also takes time.

People often ask me, "What do you eat in a day?" It's not as simple as sharing today's meals because it doesn't capture the journey that brought me here. What I eat now is the result of a gradual transition over the years. If I shared my current diet with someone just starting, it might feel overwhelming. They wouldn't see the gradual steps I took to get here. Just like building muscle at the gym, we start small and work up to our goals. Improving our diet and health follows the same principle. It's an ongoing process, not a quick fix.

Adopting a health-conscious lifestyle means we never truly finish; it becomes a way of life. There are no shortcuts. Many believe a short-term cleanse will solve their problems, but real healing takes time and consistent, sustainable habits. The better choices we make, the more they crowd out the unhealthy ones.

When transitioning to healthier choices, many worry about missing out or not fitting in. But as we progress, the foods that used to be normal no longer feel like real nourishment. I've been asked if I miss certain foods, but my mindset has changed. I don't miss foods that harm my body. Over time, through a gradual transition, our tastes and desires shift. Feeling and functioning at our best becomes our priority.

In a world filled with foods that don't truly nourish us, it's important to recognize that our health is under attack. While tempting aromas might remind us of old favorites, we learn to appreciate that our bodies deserve better. True health is a treasure, and we shouldn't settle for less.

People also ask me how I manage to avoid temptations. I'm not perfect, and I've had moments where I've strayed from my ideal diet. The key is that I don't see these foods as temptations. I've shifted my perspective – foods like meat, dairy, eggs, fried and processed foods simply aren't on my radar anymore. When I see others lining up at fast-food joints, I don't feel like I'm missing out.

In fact, I believe they're missing out on experiencing true health.

 Understanding the impact of our food choices on our health makes it easier to choose what's best for us. Over time, our tastes change, and we begin to prefer healthier options. Patience is crucial, and our transition diet paves the way for this transformation. Building health takes time and a deep understanding of our current state, which can be revealed through techniques like iridology.

 During my early health journey, I learned the importance of culinary creativity and social preparation. Food cravings arise, especially in social situations, which could lead to dietary mishaps. These cravings happen because we're used to heavy, unhealthy foods. Our lymphatic system can also harbor accumulated acids and wastes, triggering cravings as the body eliminates them.

 Cravings wane as we transition, and we naturally desire healthier foods. This process requires time and patience, as our taste buds adjust. It's important to remember that cravings are part of the transition, and choosing transitional foods is okay. For instance, I used dates and nut butter to curb my chocolate bar addiction. Over time, I transitioned to eating only the healthy dates, satisfying my sweet tooth without compromising my health.

 Transitioning is individual and takes a well-thought-out plan. It's about understanding the process and your own needs. Remember, your health is worth the effort. It's the foundation for your future, and building it requires patience, diligence, and ongoing maintenance.

Building our health requires learning to cook for ourselves during the transitional period. Unless you have a personal chef, there's no way around it. Relying on restaurants, even supposedly healthy ones, won't lead to true health. They often use oils and salts that do not promote health. Even raw vegan restaurants can lean heavily on fatty foods like nuts, seeds, and oils. It's crucial to know exactly what you're eating, and that means preparing your own food.

 If spending time in the kitchen feels extreme, you might not be ready for this step. But the good news is, there's plenty of easy-to-carry healthy options, like fruits. They're Nature's fast food, and to be honest, the simpler your choices the better!

Transitioning to healthier habits requires creativity. What works best varies for each of us. Those who succeed are usually those committed to regaining or maintaining their health. The first step is learning about mucus-forming and mucusless foods. You can find lists in Arnold Ehret's chapter 10.

A common mistake on raw or mucusless diets is underestimating the mucus-forming effects of fatty foods. All fats, including plant fats like avocados and nuts, slow digestion and healing. They're easy to overdo. Keeping fat intake around 10% of your daily diet is recommended, especially for healing. My first recommendation for anyone that wants to transition to a healthier diet is simple: eat one large meal of fruit per day and one large salad per day. Overtime the healthier foods will flood out the less-than-ideal foods.

Healthy Food Swaps

Pasta and noodles hold a special place in our hearts, and the good news is that we don't have to bid them farewell. To start, we should phase out the most mucus-forming noodle types, such as rice noodles and white flour noodles. A common transition begins with whole wheat noodles, followed by quinoa or lentil noodles, progressing to kelp noodles, and ultimately culminating in the healthiest choice of all – zucchini noodles. Crafting zucchini noodles is a breeze using an affordable handheld spiralizer. These raw zucchini noodles can be relished with a drizzle of homemade sauce, offering a mucusless, nourishing, and satisfying option. For those seeking more variety, consider crafting "coodles," or cucumber noodles. Embrace these delightful and nutritious noodles with your preferred healthy dressing or sauce and savor the flavors!

Bread, a dietary staple for many, warrants thoughtful consideration. While it may be challenging to entirely forsake bread, one can gradually reduce its consumption, reserving it for occasional cravings. When indulging in bread, opt for whole grain choices like Ezekiel bread, toasted to a crisp according to Arnold Ehret's advice. This toasting process aids in minimizing mucus-forming attributes. Enhance this choice by accompanying well-toasted bread (or any mucus-forming food) with a leafy green salad. A salad acts as a natural intestinal broom, promoting intestinal tract health and aiding elimination. Pairing bread with a leafy green salad serves an eliminative purpose. Over time, one may decide to eliminate bread entirely, a process unique to each individual based on various factors.

Burgers

Transitioning away from traditional burgers becomes a pivotal step in adopting a health-conscious diet. Conventional burgers, laden with starches, proteins, and other less-than-ideal ingredients, pose a challenge. An initial move could involve shifting towards store-bought vegan, plant-based burger options, selecting brands with minimal additives (excluding Beyond Meat). This serves as a precursor to crafting homemade plant-based burger patties. A simple approach entails baking portobello mushrooms as patties, with minimal seasoning. Alternatively, concoct burger patties from finely chopped or shredded vegetables like carrot, zucchini, mushroom, celery, and bell pepper. The challenge lies in finding an appropriate binder with low mucus-forming properties. Some may opt for a hint of mashed potato as a binder, reducing its quantity over time. For those seeking a raw alternative, dehydrated nut and vegetable-based patties offer a flavorful choice. Swap traditional buns for romaine or iceberg lettuce or consider using well-toasted bread such as Ezekiel bread. Enjoy these wholesome "burgers" with homemade raw ketchup or transition to a healthier raw sauce as desired.

Sauces and dressings add a delectable touch to meals, but commercial options often contain undesirable elements. The solution lies in creating homemade alternatives. While many store-bought sauces contain salts, vinegars, oils, preservatives, and other non-health-promoting ingredients, crafting your own empowers you to make better choices. For a mucus-free or predominantly mucus-free diet, crafting tomato-based sauces, whether raw or cooked depending on your transitional stage, serves as an excellent option. Alternatively, consider topping salads with steamed vegetables as a dressing substitute. Steamed vegetables provide adequate moisture, making them a viable dressing alternative. Embrace creative freedom in crafting your own dressings – blending a blend of carrot, bell pepper, zucchini, and other vegetables with avocado or nuts, supplemented with a hint of water. These concoctions, rich in flavor and low in fat, make for satisfying dressings. As you progress on your journey, feel free to experiment with fruit-based dressings, such as mango and lime, to add a refreshing twist. Remember, a dash of ingenuity is a valuable asset in crafting flavorful and wholesome meals.

Pizza, a beloved staple, takes the spotlight on this list due to its popularity. During my initial transition, I used whole wheat tortilla wraps as a pizza crust. Toppings like tomato sauce, pineapple, mushrooms, and peppers sufficed, as I didn't miss the absence of cheese. The realization of dairy cheese's adverse effects on health steered me away from it. Eliminating cheese, especially dairy, can be a challenge due to its addictive nature cultivated over time. While nut-based or vegan cheeses are options for transitioning, it's wise to limit processed vegan cheeses or homemade nut cheeses. These complex foods with nuts, oils, and additives might lead to digestive issues if overconsumed. Some recipes suggest alternatives like cooked and blended sweet potato with potato, although they often contain less optimal ingredients like salt and nutritional yeast. Crafting a simple cashew cheese is an option, although it won't replicate the cheese you were accustomed to. Over time, cravings for cheese wane as the body detoxifies. Avocado serves as an excellent cheese or butter substitute. Patience is key, and homemade cheese-less pizza can be both delectable and healthful!

Nice Cream

Early in my transition, I followed Arnold Ehret's dietary guidance, using cooked and raw fruits to curb artificial sweet cravings during the first year. Baked bananas with dates created a gooey, satisfying dessert, especially when paired with raw banana nice cream. This healthy treat, made by blending frozen bananas, fresh dates, and a splash of water (or other desired fruit), serves as an ideal replacement for yogurt or dairy ice cream. For a demonstration, you can find a video on making banana nice cream on my YouTube channel, "Apple Diaries." My artificial sweet cravings were appeased by dates and banana nice cream in the initial years. Today, I occasionally indulge in a substantial bowl of banana nice cream for a light dinner when a salad doesn't appeal. I strive for a well-balanced diet and aim for equal parts fruits and greens.

Tacos, once a cherished favorite, hold a special place in my heart due to my Texan heritage. Initially, I baked corn tortillas (without oil) and topped them with homemade raw or cooked tomato sauce, sautéed (in water) bell peppers, mushrooms, and jackfruit. As my diet evolved, I transitioned to using romaine lettuce as taco shells, creating flavorful lettuce boats filled with vegetables. Presently, my taco routine involves romaine lettuce boats brimming with raw greens and vegetables (shredded carrot, zucchini, bell pepper, sprouts) drizzled with a delightful raw salad dressing. As our health journey progresses, our diet naturally becomes simpler and cleaner. While there's no need to rush, moving towards a healthier direction while mastering healthy habits is essential before advancing. If dealing with chronic or degenerative conditions, a shorter transition period might be advisable due to limited time for healing.

I've comprehensively addressed the most common concerns about missing out on popular foods when transitioning to a new dietary and lifestyle approach that promotes the body's natural healing abilities. It's undeniable that the changes we make now are a response to the dietary and lifestyle choices we've made in the past, which have led to the expression of unwanted symptoms. Sadly, the prevalence of disease-forming foods in society, along with the ubiquity of fast food and junk options, complicates the transition to a Natural Human diet and lifestyle.

However, there's a silver lining: Once we establish healthier habits, they become more ingrained over time. It's normal to feel increased hunger and insatiable cravings during the initial year of transition. This can lead us to believe that fruits, greens, and vegetables will never satisfy us. Yet, understanding that this is part of the process, and that satisfaction will come with time helps navigate this stage. My personal experience echoes the sentiment that, initially, I consumed around four times the food I do today. I recognized overeating as part of the process and knew it would eventually stabilize. Most of us have spent our lives consuming complex foods that strain digestion, sapping our vital energy. Adjusting to the simple, water-rich foods that support healing takes time, as elucidated by Arnold Ehret's teachings and personal experiences.

Our mindset profoundly influences our success. An enthusiastic approach to adopting healthier eating habits and witnessing the body's self-healing fosters a smoother transition compared to those who reluctantly embrace this lifestyle due to feeling cornered. Framing the situation as others missing out on the vitality and health we're experiencing is empowering. Regrettably, many lack the chance to learn about the dietary-disease connection in this manner. Even when the information is shared, some fail to grasp its significance, perceiving it as just another diet. As the saying goes, "You can lead a horse to water, but you cannot make it drink." Don't be disheartened if family and friends don't immediately see what you do. Our responsibility is to sow seeds, disseminate information when appropriate, and wait for them to germinate. Prioritize your well-being, embark on your healing journey, and witness how everything else falls into place as a result.

Here is the recipe and instructions for the "Date/Flax Flatbread":

**Ingredients: **

- 1 cup of ground flax seeds (pre-ground in a blender or food processor)

- Half finely chopped onion (optional)

- Dried or fresh rosemary, to taste

- 1 cup of soaked dates

- Half a cup of ground sunflower seeds

**Instructions: **

1. Begin by soaking the dates to soften them. You can do this by placing the dates in a bowl of water for a few hours until they are soft and pliable.

2. Once the dates are soaked, drain them and place them in a food processor or blender.

3. Add the finely chopped onion, dried or fresh rosemary (adjust the amount to your preference), and the ground sunflower and flax seeds to the food processor.

4. Blend the ingredients together until a thick and well-mixed consistency is achieved. The mixture should hold together and not be too runny.

5. Prepare a dehydrator tray or a piece of parchment paper on a baking sheet.

6. Spread the mixture onto the parchment paper or dehydrator tray, shaping it into a thin, even layer. You can use a spatula or your hands to smooth it out.

7. Place the tray or sheet in a dehydrator or an oven set to the lowest possible temperature (usually around 105°F or 41°C).

8. Allow the flatbread to dehydrate for approximately 12 hours. Check the flatbread periodically to ensure it is drying evenly and to your desired texture.

9. Once the flatbread is fully dehydrated and has a crisp texture, remove it from the dehydrator or oven.

10. Let the flatbread cool before breaking it into desired shapes or pieces.

Enjoy your homemade date/flax flatbread as a healthier alternative to traditional bread! This flatbread is a great option for satisfying cravings and can be used in various dishes or enjoyed on its own. Remember, this recipe is customizable, so feel free to adjust the ingredients and seasonings according to your preferences.

Here is the recipe and instructions for "Raw Veggie Burgers":

**Ingredients: **
- 1 cup of walnuts (or nuts of your choice)
- 1 large carrot
- 1 stalk of celery
- 4-5 sundried tomatoes (no salt or oil)
- 2 tbsp ground flax seeds
- 1 large tomato
- 1 bell pepper

**Instructions: **

1. chop or food process walnuts, carrots, celery and pepper and set aside in a large bowl.

2. blend the tomato, sundried tomatoes and flax seeds together and mix with the other ingredients.

3. Create burger like patties and place them on the dehydrator sheets.

4. Dehydrate for approximately 4 hours, flip, and dehydrate for another 4 hours.

Enjoy these burgers on their own, in a salad or use iceberg lettuce or collard wraps for a healthy bun alternative.

Here is the recipe and instructions for "homemade raw ketchup":

**Ingredients: **

- 1-2 large tomatoes

- 3-4 dates

- ½ cup of sundried tomatoes

**Instructions: **

1. Blend all three ingredients together.

This makes a thick "ketchup like" sauce to top the "raw burgers with".

Here is the recipe and instructions for "Mango Vinaigrette":

**Ingredients: **

- 1 large mango (can use frozen equivalent)

- 1 tbsp of Apple Cider Vinegar (I use lemon juice instead)

- 1 tbsp of Coconut Amino's

- ½ tsp smoked paprika

- ½ cup of water

**Instructions: **

1. Blend all ingredients together and enjoy.

This makes a delicious creamy salad dressing.

Here is the recipe and instructions for "Sweet and Sour Dressing":

**Ingredients: **

- 6 dates
- juice of one whole lemon
- ½ tsp of smoked paprika (optional)
- ½ tsp of Apple Cider Vinegar
- little water
- half a small zucchini

**Instructions: **

1. Blend all ingredients together and enjoy.

Here is the recipe and instructions for "Orange Dressing":

**Ingredients: **

- 2 cups of freshly squeezed orange juice
- 1 cup of cashews
- small handful of parsley
- 1 tsp of dulce

**Instructions: **

Blend all ingredients together and enjoy.

Here is the recipe and instructions for "My Raw Wraps":

**Ingredients: **

- 2 large carrots

- 10 dates

- 1 cup water

- ½ tsp smoked paprika

- ½ cup of ground flax

**Instructions: **

Grind flax seeds in the blender if they are whole flax seeds.

Add rough chopped carrots, dates, water, paprika to the flax seeds and blend.

Once a smooth consistency divide the batter into 4 small piles on dehydrator trays lined with parchment or silicone.

Using a spatula, create small circular wraps about ¼ inch thick.

Pop trays into the dehydrator.

Dehydrate for approximately 4-5 hours.

Flip the wraps upside down, peel off parchment paper and dehydrate on the other side for another hour or two.

Remove wraps and fill with greens, tomato and my "Cashew Lemon Dressing".

Here is the recipe and instructions for "Cashew Lemon Dressing":

**Ingredients: **

- Handful of cashews

- The juice of 1 whole lemon

- 6 small dates

- ½ tsp smoked paprika

- ½ cup of water

- A small piece of zucchini

- A small piece of carrot

**Instructions: **

Blend all ingredients together and enjoy.

Some people prefer to soak the cashews for approximately 3 hours before draining and blending but it is not necessary. This sauce is sweet, tangy and goes well with tomatoes and spinach stuffed into my "Raw Wraps" recipe.

Chapter 13
Steps Towards Health and Healing

When you know the truth, you'll know what to do. There's no one-size-fits-all answer for transitioning to better health because it varies for each person due to various factors and levels of understanding. But knowing the truth simplifies it.

You might be wondering how to improve your health. Well, health and healing are closely linked. The diet that maintains good health is the same one that sets the stage for the body to heal itself. Some people claim that fruit is only good for the short term and healing but not for long-term health, which is contradictory. If it's healthy, it's healthy; there's no in-between. This confusion stems from conflicting information out there.

It's unfortunate that many people discover this path when their health is already suffering, after trying various treatments and methods that didn't help. They might be better off not doing anything at all. I faced a similar situation and had to find my own way when traditional methods failed me.

It's challenging for many to accept that we're designed for simple, natural foods only like fruits, greens, vegetables, nuts and seeds. So why did we diverge from our natural diet? There are theories, but the truth remains elusive. Perhaps desperation or outside influence led to the consumption of animal products and cooked foods. What we do know for sure is that we're meant to eat foods that grow in nature in their raw form.

I can personally vouch for the benefits of a diet based on raw plant foods after trying other diets without success. Some might dismiss my experience as anecdotal, but the truth often seems simple when we step back and examine our habits.

My top suggestion for health and healing is to examine your current diet and lifestyle and make changes. Sometimes, a few unhealthy habits or dietary preferences are at the root of health issues, even if you have some healthy habits too.

Many people underestimate the impact of simple suggestions on their overall health. We tend to favor complexity, but every daily choice accumulates and affects our health. For instance, taking time to rest your mind daily can help restore nerve energy, which is essential for health maintenance and healing. Accumulating healthy habits over time is crucial for overall health.

So, when someone claims they never get sick, it might indicate a lack of nerve energy to initiate a cleansing event, which could lead to chronic health issues in the long run.

We must learn which foods promote health and which ones deteriorate our health over time. Health-promoting foods are hydrating, while non-health-promoting foods are dehydrating. Once I learned the truth about meat and dairy consumption, I couldn't enjoy eating them anymore, making it easy to eliminate them from my diet. I recommend reading books like Dr. Robert Morse's "Detox Miracle Sourcebook" and Arnold Ehret's "Rational Fasting" for in-depth insights into the harmful effects of meat and dairy.

These animal products are acidic, lowering our body's pH and causing inflammation and tissue damage. They also lead to toxin buildup, provide an ideal environment for parasites, hinder cellular respiration, damage adrenal glands, and contribute to chronic fatigue. Meat is a stimulant and can disrupt our blood's pH balance, leading to weakened bones over time.

Change doesn't happen overnight; it's a slow process, just like how poor health develops gradually through small violations against our well-being. Conversely, building good health also takes time and happens through consistent, health-promoting choices.

It's evident that eliminating meat, dairy, and all animal products is essential for health and healing.

Now, can you guess which food is the absolute worst for human health? It's safe to assume that most people are aware that processed foods, fast food, and items with long lists of ingredients are detrimental to health. The more ingredients a food has, the worse it is for your well-being. Real food doesn't need a list of ingredients. A good starting point is to incorporate a large salad and a large fruit meal (or a freshly made juice/smoothie) into your daily routine. This leaves less room for non-health-promoting foods while improving hydration.

While juicing or blending isn't the most natural practice, it can help those in need of change and gradually reduce the intake of unhealthy foods. Daily juicing or smoothies can improve hydration levels and correct chronic dehydration, which many people suffer from unknowingly.

Over time, as the daily salad and fruit routine becomes a habit, your body will crave healthier foods, and your taste buds will adapt. It takes motivation, time, and patience in the beginning.

Now, let's return to the steps you can take for the body to heal itself. But before that, let me share some foundational information from Lauren Whiteman, who, along with Nat Farris and I, runs a monthly subscription "Terrain Diet Support Group" on Facebook. We are passionate about sharing the health-saving information we've learned through Natural Hygiene principles and are dedicated to helping others on their health journeys. Here's what Lauren wrote, which sets the stage for the steps to follow.

Disease is not a sudden mystery or accident. Many people think of disease as something that strikes out of the blue, with no prior warnings. However, the truth is that disease begins long before it's diagnosed, often in childhood.

From infancy, we are exposed to foods that may cause discomfort but are unaware of how to communicate our pain. Our parents feed us acidic breast milk or toxic formulas, along with other processed and animal-based foods. These early dietary choices set the stage for our health.

Layer by layer, toxins accumulate in our bodies, and we experience symptoms like rashes, colds, and fevers. These are warning signs of the body's distress, but we continue to consume harmful foods.

As we grow older, we might experience acne, headaches, fatigue and a need for stimulants like coffee or sugar. Our energy declines, and we blame it on "normal aging," but it's not normal at all.

Disease is a progressive process, building over time with each meal of cooked, processed, and denatured foods. Conversely, health can be achieved progressively by eliminating these harmful foods and supplying our bodies with what they truly need.

The key is to listen to our bodies, recognize the warnings, and make changes. Disease is not an accident; it's the result of years of mistakes in our lifestyle and diet. However, it's entirely within our control to reverse it by learning and eliminating these mistakes.

If you're ready to make changes and need support or motivation, consider joining a support and education group like the 30-Day Terrain Model Diet Support and Education Group.

I hope Lauren's explanation helped you understand why people get sick and why it's essential to have the right knowledge for healing. Many people suffer because they lack this knowledge, and it's unfortunate that this life-saving information is often buried under misinformation.

Now, let's talk about the steps for health and healing:

1. **Know Your Species:** We are frugivores, designed to eat fruits and raw greens. It's crucial to understand our biological nature and transition to our species-appropriate diet gradually.

2. **Understand Cause and Effect:** Disease doesn't happen by accident. It's the result of our daily dietary and lifestyle choices over time. Our health today reflects our past choices.

3. **Eliminate Harmful Foods:** Start by removing processed, fried, fast food, and all dairy products from your diet. Dairy is highly mucus-forming and addictive.

4. **Incorporate Healthy Habits:** Begin with two daily habits: replace your first meal with fresh fruit or a smoothie and have a large leafy green salad with your evening meal.

5. **Stay Hydrated:** Drink plenty of water, up to a gallon or more daily, especially when transitioning to a diet rich in raw fruits and vegetables.

6. **Ditch Animal Products:** Remove all meat and eggs from your diet. Explore healthy alternatives like scrambled zucchini or tofu as substitutes.

7. **Embrace Plant-Based Staples:** Make raw fruit, leafy greens, and raw veggies your main foods. Over time, your body will adapt to love them. It's important to eat enough of the correct foods to avoid cravings for less-than-ideal foods.

8. **Review Your Diet:** Gradually eliminate less-than-ideal foods like rice, grains, or beans. Pair these foods with a leafy green salad when you do eat them.

9. **Continuous Improvement:** The transition diet is about refining your choices as you go. Stay committed to your health goals, and you'll achieve them over time.

Remember that health and healing are intertwined, and the diet that maintains health is the same one that supports the body in healing itself. It's not a separate process. Healthy living and dietary choices are essential, and they work together for a holistic approach to well-being. Once you experience the benefits of good health, you'll never be misled again.

Let's talk about more changes we can make to improve our health. There's a rumor that fruit is only good for short-term health and healing, but not for the long term. It sounds strange, right? But people are often confused about health because there's so much conflicting information out there.

Many folks discover this kind of information when they're already suffering and have tried many other things that didn't work. They may have gone to doctors, tried various treatments, taken pills, and even had surgeries, all with no real improvement. It can be a last resort for some.

Ideally, people should learn about this before their bodies start showing symptoms. It's easier to make these dietary and lifestyle changes when you're not forced to by your body's distress signals.

Now, why did humanity stray so far from its natural diet? Why did we start eating animals and their products if it's not our natural food? There are many theories, but no one knows for sure. It might have been due to a major event, like climate change or war, forcing people to adapt to new diets. We can't be certain about the exact reasons.

One thing we can be sure of is that our bodies are designed for simple, raw foods like fruits, greens, vegetables, nuts, and seeds. I know this because I tried different diets, including one with organic animal products, for years, and my health kept declining. It was only when I radically changed my diet, eliminating animal products and adopting a health-promoting one, that I finally found relief.

Some might dismiss my experience as anecdotal, but that's okay. Changing your diet, especially when you're used to certain foods, can be scary. But often, the truth is simple. If you want to understand the cause of your health issues, look at your diet and lifestyle over the past 10-20 years. Changing these habits can make a big difference. Also, remember that past trauma can play a role in your health, so it's important to address that too.

Now, I'll talk about some simple practices that may not seem like a big deal but can have a significant impact on your health. What we consume regularly affects our overall health. Our past habits and choices add up over time, shaping who we are today. Let me give you an example: our body has a limited supply of nerve energy throughout our lifetime. Unhealthy dietary and lifestyle choices, prolonged stressful situations, pharmaceutical use, and other habits can deplete this energy. To restore this nerve energy, consider closing your eyes daily for at least 10 minutes. This practice helps your body repair and rejuvenate. It's a moment of rest that can accumulate positive effects on your overall health. Over time, with this practice and a health-promoting diet, your body can store enough nerve energy to initiate healing or cleansing processes, like cold or flu symptoms, to detoxify.

Children tend to get sick more often because they haven't depleted their nerve energy like adults have. When someone who clearly doesn't take care of themselves claims they "never get sick," it's a red flag. It often means their body lacks the energy to even initiate cleansing events (sickness), leading to the accumulation of toxins.

Understanding which foods promote health and which degrade it is crucial. Health-promoting foods are hydrating, while non-health-promoting ones are often dehydrating. Once you learn the truth about meat and dairy consumption, it can be hard to enjoy those foods again. They may even become effortless to eliminate from your diet. Animal products inflict pain and torture on animals, and they harm human health. Meat and dairy are acidic, leading to inflammation and tissue damage, lowering our body's pH, and weakening bones. They also contain hormones, steroids, and neurotransmitters that damage our adrenal glands and cause chronic fatigue.

Changing your diet can take time, as nothing happens overnight. Just as poor health builds up slowly, good health builds up through small, health-promoting choices and habits over time.

Processed foods, fast food, and fried or oily foods are among the first things to eliminate from your diet. Real food doesn't have a long list of ingredients. Start by incorporating a large salad and a fruit meal each day, ideally having fruit as your first meal on an empty stomach. Fruit digests quickly and provides hydration after a night's rest. Drinking more water, ideally a gallon to a gallon and a half daily, is essential.

After eliminating processed and oily foods, the next step is to remove all dairy products from your diet. They are mucus-forming and not meant for human consumption.

Grounding, or earthing, is a practice with numerous health benefits. It involves direct contact with the Earth's surface, which is negatively charged. We are positively charged, so grounding helps us take up negative ions, neutralizing positive charges from things like radio waves, stress, or exercise. You can ground by walking barefoot outside or using earthing sheets for sleeping.

Sunlight exposure is another underrated health factor. The chemistry of our blood is influenced by sunlight, making it crucial for overall health. Regular sunlight strengthens our skin, organs, and glands. It's vital to get enough sunlight, especially in today's world where it can be hard to come by. So, take advantage of sunny days when you can, as sunlight benefits various aspects of our health.

Let's talk about sunglasses and why wearing them can harm your health. Sunglasses block certain wavelengths of sunlight from reaching your retinas, which can affect your body's ability to produce vitamin D (which is actually a hormone, not a vitamin). Some people use "light sensitivity" as a reason to wear sunglasses, but as you adopt a healthy plant and fruit-based diet, you may find that light sensitivity (often a sign of a weak, toxic liver) diminishes as your organs and glands heal and strengthen.

Now, let's touch on the harmful effects of sunscreen. What you put on your skin can be absorbed into your bloodstream, so if you wouldn't eat it, you probably shouldn't slather it on your skin. Moreover, the chemicals and unnatural ingredients found in most sunscreens end up in our waterways and harm the environment. Using sunscreen can also interfere with sweating, breathing, and melatonin production. True "sunscreen" can be found in your diet. Eating healthier enables your body to cleanse itself of internal waste, making you less prone to sunburn. Our relationship with the sun can be beautiful if we align with natural laws and eat in harmony with our design. Acidic individuals who regularly consume acid-forming, mucus-forming foods are more susceptible to sunburn.

When you've had enough sun for the day, simply protect yourself by wearing a hat or light clothing. As an alternative to commercial moisturizers, you can use the juice from melons or grapes you're eating as a natural, edible moisturizer or after-sun care.

Now, let's briefly discuss a couple of non-health promoting practices that many of us engage in without much thought. Body piercings, for instance, can block energy flow over time, which may lead to discomfort and a sense of rejection by your body. Removing piercings can bring a feeling of freedom. Tattoos, on the other hand, introduce ink toxicity to your body, which can have adverse effects on your health. Knowing what you know now, you might reconsider these practices.

Intermittent fasting, like skipping breakfast, can have positive health effects over time. Some people may find it challenging to give up their early morning meal right away, and that's okay. It's essential to establish healthy eating habits before diving into fasting. Over time, as you make fruit your first meal, you may naturally delay it to provide your digestive system with more rest in the morning. This extended fasting period can help your body heal and address internal issues more effectively. Remember that your body can focus on only one complex task at a time, so when it's digesting food, it's not healing. By gradually extending your fasting window, you can experience the health benefits without feeling deprived or uncomfortable.

Creating a healthy home environment is also crucial. Avoid using toxic cleaning supplies and products. Opt for natural alternatives like vinegar, baking soda, or natural dish soap for cleaning. When it comes to laundry, choose a natural detergent or simply use baking soda. You might even find that you need less soap on your skin; water can often suffice. Using a natural, preservative-free shampoo can also make a difference. You may only need to shampoo your hair every 7-10 days, and over time, your scalp's health can improve, reducing issues like itching and flakiness.

Now, let's talk about some health and beauty practices you might reconsider. Highlighting your hair with chemicals can damage it over time. Instead, let the sun naturally give your hair highlights, which can be even better. Tattoos, unfortunately, can contribute to heavy metal poisoning due to the inorganic, heavy metals found in tattoo ink. The continuous needle pricks, pain, and trauma to the skin from tattoos can also cause damage. Nail polish and nail polish remover contain toxic chemicals like formaldehyde, toluene, and dibutyl phthalate (DBP). These chemicals have been associated with various health issues and are banned in some countries. Lastly, working in a nail or hair salon can expose you to these harmful chemicals, highlighting the importance of choosing safer alternatives.

I didn't use much makeup, but as I learned about the chemicals in makeup, I stopped using most of it. I believe in letting my skin breathe, so I avoid covering it with makeup, face creams, or powders. It took me a couple of years to get comfortable without applying moisturizer, which I once used regularly. Instead, I started using fresh aloe vera, but later, I learned it might not be good for the skin. So, I began using fruit juice from grapes or melons, which works great as a moisturizer. Healthy, hydrated skin comes from within, so trying to fix dry skin with external products is just a temporary solution. Wrinkles are often caused by dehydration, so a diet rich in fruits and leafy greens can help improve your skin over time.

Another important aspect of health is staying hydrated. Finding truly clean and uncontaminated water can be challenging, but I believe distilled water is a good option. It's essential to drink enough water daily, especially if you've had a history of dehydrating foods. Mineral and spring water can contain inorganic minerals that may lead to issues like kidney stones. I prefer distillation because it creates pure water similar to rainwater. Distilled water has a pH of 6.0 and can help flush out inorganic minerals, promoting overall health. Claims about the benefits of alkaline water are not convincing to me because the stomach is acidic, and too much alkaline water can dilute digestive juices. It's important to differentiate between inorganic and organic minerals, as distilled water can help remove inorganic minerals from the body.

Rest is another vital aspect of health. Your body won't oversleep; it will rest as much as it needs. Poor sleep patterns and digestive disturbances are often related. To improve sleep, avoid eating too close to bedtime, ideally stopping at least 3 hours before sleep. Restful sleep can be challenging when you're in poor health, but it improves as your health does. If you struggle with sleep, try closing your eyes for at least 10 minutes daily to restore vital nerve energy. This practice can have positive effects on your overall health, even though it may seem simple at first. Give it a few months, and you'll notice the benefits.

In summary, I leave you with these 10 simple tips for better health:

1. **Limit Screen Time**: Reduce your exposure to blue light from devices like cell phones and computers. You can set your Wi-Fi to turn off at a specific time each night and try to avoid screens after 8 pm.

2. **Fresh Air and Ventilation**: Make sure to sleep in a well-ventilated room and get plenty of fresh air. Remember, the air we breathe is a crucial nutrient for our bodies.

3. **Exercise Wisely**: Be mindful of when and how you exercise. When transitioning to a healthier diet, your energy levels may drop initially. It's essential to listen to your body and not push too hard. Gradually build your stamina and strength as your body adjusts.

4. **Hydration is Key**: Focus on staying hydrated. Drinking clean, pure water is vital for your health. Distilled water can be an excellent choice as it helps eliminate inorganic minerals from your body.

5. **Rest and Sleep**: Get enough rest and quality sleep. Your body will naturally rest for the time it needs when you're in good health. Avoid eating too close to bedtime to improve sleep quality.

6. **Health Takes Time**: Understand that achieving optimal health is a process. It took time to develop poor health, and it will take time to build it back up. Be patient with yourself and allow your body to heal and adapt.

7. **Live by Example**: Lead by example and let the improvements in your health and life speak for themselves. When others see the positive changes in you, they'll be more inclined to consider a healthy lifestyle.

8. **Learn and Educate**: Educate yourself about the cleansing and healing stages your body goes through as you adopt a healthier lifestyle. This knowledge will help you stay committed during challenging times and counter misconceptions about your diet.

9. **No Deficiency, Just Healing**: Don't worry about deficiencies. If someone on a high-fruit, greens, nuts/seeds, and raw vegetable diet appears depleted, it's likely due to a congested lymphatic system. Healing takes time, and a skinny period can be part of the process. Understand that it's a normal part of healing, not a sign of deficiency.

10. **Be a Healthy Example**: Live a healthy lifestyle for yourself and set an example for others. In a world filled with tempting and convenient but unhealthy foods, being a positive example can inspire others to choose a healthier path.

Remember, health is a journey, not a destination, and each step you take toward better health is a step in the right direction.

Chapter 14
A Collection of Inspiring Quotes

I'm devoting this chapter to my favorite quotes because I really love them. Quotes are like tiny treasures that can teach us a lot in just a few words. I've been collecting these valuable quotes for a long time, and now I'm excited to share them all in my very first book!

I hope you like these quotes as much as I do. Whenever I feel uninspired, I read them again, and they always make me think and motivate me.

1. "You don't need treatment. The fever, inflammation, coughing, etc., constitute the healing process. Just get out of their way and permit them to complete their work. Don't try to 'aid' nature. She doesn't need your puny aid—she only asks that you cease interfering."

   – Herbert Shelton

2. "Cutting out bad habits is far more effective than cutting out organs."

   – Herbert Shelton

3. "If you desire to truly live, you will cease trying to find magic tricks and shortcuts to life and learn the simple laws of being and order your life in conformity with these. Realign your life with the laws of nature—this and this alone constitutes living to live."

   – Herbert Shelton

4. "Old age is not a time of life. It is a condition of the body. It is

not time that ages the body, it is abuse that does."

  - Herbert Shelton

5. "Although man has included meat in his diet for thousands of years, his anatomy and physiology, and the chemistry of his digestive juices, are still unmistakably those of a frugivorous animal."

  - Herbert Shelton

6. "The so-called symptoms of disease are manifestations of an inherent principle of the organism to restore healthy function and to resist offending agents and influences."

  - Herbert Shelton

7. "In our present day of enlightenment, it should not require much in a way of argument or illustration, for all people to readily recognize that our bodies are what they are, as a result of what they feed upon. Now, what does your body feed upon?"

  - Van R. Wilcox, author of "Correct Living"

8. "Most men can understand eating to get strong, but it takes a long time to educate them to stop eating to get strong."

  - Dr. Tilden

9. "It is disease that saves life. It is disease that actually cures the body. By means of disease, poisons are eliminated, which might have caused death, had they been allowed to remain."

  - Bernarr Macfadden

10. "The doctor of the future will give us no medicine but will interest his patients in the care of the human frame, in diet and in

the cause and prevention of disease."

   - Thomas Edison

11. "There can be only one permanent revolution – a moral one; the regeneration of the inner man. How is this revolution to take place? Nobody knows how it will take place in humanity, but every man feels it clearly in himself. And yet in our world everybody thinks of changing humanity, and nobody thinks of changing himself."

   - Leo Tolstoy

12. "Health and, in turn, 'freedom' is an inside job."

   - Maria Manazza

13. "True healing is not a 'quick fix' but a regeneration that comes from removing all waste from the body."

   - Professor Arnold Ehret

14. "Disease is a fermentation and decay-process of body substances or of surplus and unnatural food material which, in the course of time, has accumulated, especially in the digestive organs, and which makes its appearance in the shape of mucus excretion."

   - Professor Arnold Ehret

15. "Health or Disease is a choice. The current state of one's healt is the summation of all our daily dietary/lifestyle choices to date

   - Maria Manazza

16. "Think about your dietary/lifestyle choices in depth because your quality of life depends on you being correct in those choices."

   - Maria Manazza

17. "As cravings arise, understand that they are only the expression of poisons that are circulating through your bloodstream. You are not your addiction to mucus, and over time as those poisons dissipate, you will no longer crave the foods that cause harm to your body."

   - Professor Spira

18. "We do not have 'health-related issues,' we have dietary, pharmaceutical & lifestyle related issues."

   - Maria Manazza

19. "No one can overcome a health problem using the same mindset that created the problem."

   - Thomas Edison

20. "In health, there is no disease. You do not find cancer in healthy tissue."

   - Robert Morse, N.D.

21. "There is no magic or mystery to health or disease. Disease is a natural process! When we understand how the body works, and what causes the tissues in the body to fail, we will then understand what causes disease symptoms, and how to reverse it."

- Robert Morse, N.D.

22. "The greatest discovery ever made in our knowledge of healing was not the discovery of the alleged healing properties of some noxious weed or of the curative virtue of fungi or mineral poisons, but that the remedial power resides in the living organism and not in the things extrinsic to it."

- "Rubies in the Sand (The Myth of Medicine)" by Herbert M Shelton

23. "Nature does not hurry yet everything is accomplished."

- Lao Tzu

24. "Although man has included meat in his diet for thousands of years, his anatomy and physiology, and the chemistry of his digestive juices, are still unmistakably those of a frugivorous animal."

- Herbert Shelton

25. "Disease is not caught, and disease is not mysterious. Disease is developed, built & created through daily accumulations that reflect our choices over time."

- Maria Manazza

26. "The solution for pollution is dilution."

- Lauren Whiteman

27. "'Tis better to be ignorant than to know so much that isn't so."

- TC Fry

28. "Life should be built on the conservation of energy."

   – Herbert Shelton

29. "Everyone is so afraid of feeling bad when in reality we must feel bad at times to heal."

   – Maria Manazza

30. "Diseases are simply signs & symptoms that reflect that the body is not being provided with the correct conditions for health."

   – Maria Manazza

I was thinking about a quote by TC. Fry on saving energy. During my walk today, I thought that if I were to put it simply, I'd say, "Life should be about using energy wisely." Saving energy is crucial, but it's also important to spend some energy on healthy activities like exercising, having fun, and being happy.

Chapter 15
Health Concerns Simplified

Our world is full of complicated science about food, and it is making people confused about what is healthy. Nowadays, some folks even need scientific studies to prove that eating raw fruits and vegetables is good for them! Here are some frequent questions that people on a healthy, raw, fruit-based diet need to answer. If they cannot, others might doubt their choice. I do not mean to be negative towards curious folks, because we are all influenced by the same ideas. These questions keep coming up when people learn about our diet, year after year. So, I have put together quick answers to help people save time and avoid frustration.

The Great Protein Myth

"Where do you get your protein?"

The "Great Protein Myth" has led many people to harm their health, thinking they were doing the right thing. Eating too much high-protein food is a major cause of diseases in humans. Surprisingly, even after this myth has been proven false, nutrition and industry experts still promote these outdated and harmful ideas. Consuming too much protein causes health problems, even though many still believe the opposite.

Protein is not the body's main fuel, as many mistakenly think. Our bodies run on simple sugars. Complex proteins turn into acids, which can harm our cells. Animal proteins can putrefy inside us, causing body odor and bad breath. We humans are meant to eat mostly fruits and veggies, not lots of protein, especially from animals. High protein diets make our livers produce extra cholesterol, leading to issues like gallstones and kidney problems. Too much protein causes inflammation, swelling, and can even lead to tumors and organ failure. Most diseases can be linked back to eating too much protein.

The truth is our bodies do not need complete proteins. There is no such thing as a "protein deficiency" that can kill you. What our bodies really need are amino acids, the basic building blocks of protein, so we can make our own. When we eat animal proteins, our bodies cannot recognize them, and it causes problems.

Meat is stimulating, irritating, and inflammatory for our bodies. We are not built to eat animal proteins. Plus, animals raised on factory farms carry a lot of harmful stuff like antibiotics, vaccines, and hormones. Eating meat means consuming pain and suffering.

That is the basic idea of why high-protein diets are bad for our health. If you want more info, you can check out Dr. Morse's Detox Miracle Sourcebook or read about it in "*The Science and Fine Art of Food and Nutrition*" by Herbert Shelton, especially Chapter 13. You can also listen to experts like Dr. Milton Mills and Dr. Brooke Goldner, M.D., who talk about this topic. Many plant-based doctors and health enthusiasts share valuable information on this subject too.

Fruit and Sugar: Is It Too Much?

No, fruit does not have too much sugar. Nature does not make mistakes. It is just that schools, science, and doctors have told us to limit sugar for assorted reasons like losing weight and managing diabetes. This misinformation makes people scared of one of the healthiest food groups. It is strange that they put fruit sugar (fructose) in the same category as unhealthy sugars like processed and complex sugars. Fructose is a simple sugar, our body's natural fuel, essential for good health. It is crucial for our brain and cells. Science studying fructose on its own is odd because we usually eat whole fruits with fiber, fat, etc. To put it simply, fruit sugar is a simple, healthy sugar that fuels our body. Fructose metabolizes better than other sugars, making it suitable for type 1 diabetics because it does not need insulin like other sugars do.

Do All Fruitarians Have Teeth Problems?

Tooth problems can happen with people who mostly eat fruit, but it is not an absolute rule. Some fruitarians make common mistakes that can mislead others. It is important to know that the fruit itself is not the issue. Ripe fruit does not cause health problems; it is one of our natural foods. Teeth problems tend to occur when fruitarians eat only fruit, neglecting leafy greens, raw veggies, and nuts/seeds. They often juice and blend fruit instead of eating it whole. Some groups even advise skipping leafy greens, claiming they slow down healing. Greens take a bit longer to digest, but they are crucial. Chewing greens builds strong teeth and jaw muscles, aids digestion, and provides essential minerals. Long juice cleanses without chewing, greens, or fiber can lead to teeth problems. Our teeth reflect our overall health and are connected to our organs through blood vessels and nerves. Teeth issues are not just about brushing; they indicate inner problems. In today's world, we eat soft foods and smoothies, giving our teeth little exercise. Fruit does not harm our teeth; it is foods like grains and refined sugars that are the real culprits. Our natural diet does not cause tooth decay, but not eating what is right for our species or ignoring greens can have consequences. Remember, "Use it, or Lose it" applies to teeth too, they need exercise!

Vegans and B12: Is Deficiency Common?

Let me start by clearing something up: B12 deficiency is not exclusive to vegans; it affects meat eaters too. However, the focus is on plant eaters, for marketing reasons. B12 comes from our gut bacteria, so taking supplements will not really fix the issue. Supplements burden the body and do not create the right conditions for self-healing. If someone is low on B12 or other nutrients, they need to clean up their body by returning to a natural diet to allow it to heal and recover. There are no quick fixes for health problems that took years to develop, even though the supplement industry might make you believe it. You cannot just take a B12 vitamin and expect it to fix problems caused by waste buildup and compromised gut health. People often do not want to give up herbs, supplements, stimulants, processed foods, and unnatural substances. They do not want to wait for the body to heal, which requires patience and going through uncomfortable periods as it detoxifies. Healing means going through highs and lows.

What About Weight Loss? I Don't Want to Get Too Thin.

Focusing on weight should not be the main concern when adopting this diet/lifestyle. If fear of getting too thin is the primary worry, it shows a lack of understanding of the process. Even if you become "too skinny" by others' standards, your body will balance itself over time as you provide the right conditions for healing. Mainstream messages try to normalize being overweight or over nourished for profit, but your body is always working to maintain health. If your body is full of acids and waste and starts releasing some, you might go through a skinny phase. This phase is not avoidable; it is nature's way. Some people eat more fat to prevent further weight loss, but it only delays the inevitable and does not solve the problem. Our species needs some fat, but too much creates issues, like blocking absorption and producing excess mucus. Ideally, our diet should have less than 10% fat. Rapid weight loss despite consuming enough calories can happen due to malabsorption, which is common. If you do not let this period derail you and continue with a natural diet, your body will correct itself. However, not everyone is confident enough to go through this process, so they return to their old habits, thinking that it is healthy. It is not; it is familiar. Some claim that they tried a natural diet but became too skinny and weak, so they went back to meat or other non-natural foods. They misinterpret what is happening. Understanding the process means accepting periods of hardship, like becoming too skinny for a while or dealing with uncomfortable detox symptoms. I experienced the skinny phase for about eight months to a year. People commented on my weight and advised me to eat meat, but today my weight is stable, and I am not too skinny. Sometimes people gain water weight when they switch to a natural diet because their body is dehydrated and wants to dilute the acids. Weight can fluctuate as the body adjusts to healthier dietary changes, but patience and understanding are essential because this path requires time to sweep out years of accumulated waste from unnatural food choices.

Are Nightshade Foods Bad for You?

Nightshade vegetables and fruits, when eaten raw, are healthy. Some nightshades, like potatoes, need to be cooked to be edible. Our bodies have a natural way of recognizing if a food is not healthy through its taste, like spiciness or bitterness. However, it is often us humans who ignore these signals and eat them anyway. Healthy nightshades include raw foods like tomatoes and bell peppers, which are usually fine for most people. If someone experiences negative symptoms from consuming these health-promoting nightshades in their raw, whole form, it often indicates underlying health issues. It is important to note that people also report "allergies" to other healthy foods like watermelon, mangoes, or strawberries. It is not the food's fault; these foods are not toxic for some humans and healthy for others. People who clean up their diets and heal often find that their allergy issues with these foods disappear.

Why Are There Ex-Vegans?

When people ask about ex-vegans, it shows they might not understand the difference between a "Vegan" diet and eating what we are biologically designed to eat. "Vegan" is not a specific diet; it is an ethical stance against animal exploitation. Ten vegans can have completely different diets, and there are both healthy and unhealthy foods within the vegan spectrum. Some vegans prioritize ethics over health and might not make the healthiest food choices, leading to feeling worse than when they ate meat. Processed vegan products can be unhealthy, filled with chemicals and preservatives. Some people return to eating meat and animal products because they did not have the correct dietary information to maintain health and mistakenly believed they had no other option. Diverse types of vegans exist, such as whole food vegans, raw vegans, whole-food plant-based vegans, and many more. Whole food vegans focus on plant-based diets, often following guidelines from plant-based doctors. While this diet can help, it may not lead to optimal health overall. Doctors may recommend minimizing fruit intake due to sugar concerns, which can be misleading. Some may not emphasize the importance of hydration. While these diets are healthier than many others, they may not align with our species' natural diet. Everyone has the freedom to choose how far they want to take their dietary changes. It is crucial to understand our species-appropriate diet to make educated decisions about our health. Some may remain in the middle ground, and that is perfectly fine. The healing journey involves patience, understanding, and trial and error. Successful healing requires persistence, going through pain without suppressing it, and learning about the health and healing process to be prepared for unexpected challenges.

I just wanted to mention that the path towards health and healing is filled with plenty of ups and downs and trial and error. Any person that has successfully healed their health issues will tell you this, but the difference between success and failure on this path is that those individuals that are successful in their health endeavors did not give up when they hit a roadblock or when things got uncomfortable, they just got back at it. They were also willing to go through pain because going through pain is part of the healing process and there is no suppressing that pain or numbing that pain with anything. Those who are successful also take the time to learn all that they can about the health and healing process so that they can be prepared for the unexpected instead of relying on someone else to tell them if what they are experiencing is normal or not. Every headache that I experienced as a cleansing symptom (instead of from my past less than ideal choices) did not derail me from this path, I would tell myself that the headache that I was experiencing could very well be the last headache that I would ever experience again because I knew that it was only a matter of time before my body healed completely. Over time my re- occurring headaches became less frequent and less severe until I was finally headache free, but it was not easy. I will note that it was not until I transitioned to a 100% raw food diet that my headache issue finally resolved. The headaches would still occur from time to time while I was eating 80% raw while including some steamed vegetables, or baked veggies in my diet.

This concludes the most common health concerns that tend to surface for those that go on to adopting healthier diets devoid of animal products and meat. It's not easy for people to change their diet without facing challenges and various levels of scrutiny from others. But no matter what some of these bizarre scientists and doctors say, most people innately know that raw fruit and whole fresh raw foods are health promoting even if they have no plans of taking that route themselves.

When we start eating healthier, it's common to experience cleansing and healing symptoms. These symptoms might make us seek quick fixes from doctors or natural remedies, but this keeps us stuck in a cycle of symptom suppression. To truly heal, we need to understand and embrace these symptoms instead of trying to avoid them.

Cleansing symptoms can be frustrating because we expect to feel amazing right away when we switch to a healthier diet. We wonder why we do not feel great immediately. This impatience can make us question if we are on the right path.

But healing does not happen in a straight line. The body goes through ups and downs as it heals, and this is a natural part of the process. There is no set timeline for how long healing will take because it varies for each person. However, when we adopt our natural diet as a permanent lifestyle, the healing journey becomes less about the time it takes and more about our overall well-being.

It is also about how you see things. Those who embrace this lifestyle and genuinely enjoy the foods they eat tend to succeed. Being okay with standing out from the crowd is important too. That's why waiting until serious health problems arise before making the switch isn't ideal. People forced into this lifestyle due to failing health may resist it more than those who choose it proactively.

Your perspective matters a lot. Personally, I have never enjoyed food more than I do now because it's not only delicious but also nourishing. Building health takes time, so we should not stress about every single issue or symptom that arises when we align with our natural diet.

I help run a group called the *"Terrain Diet Support Group,"* and based on years of consultations, I can confidently say that experiencing cleansing symptoms is quite common and usually not a cause for concern unless they're causing extreme pain that's unbearable.

What are some common cleansing symptoms people experience?

Tiredness and Lethargy: Feeling drained of energy is typical when transitioning to a natural diet. The body is directing energy towards healing.

Weakness: Alongside tiredness, you might feel physically weaker as your body detoxifies and heals.

3. **Dizziness:** Buildup of waste in the inner ear can lead to dizziness, though it can be unsettling.

4. **Dry Skin:** Skin dryness can result from the elimination of acids through the skin, a natural process that requires patience.

5. **Phlegm/Mucus:** The body expels mucus and phlegm containing toxins as it cleanses itself.

6. **Cold/Flu-like Symptoms:** These symptoms can arise as the body releases stored toxins, and it's part of the healing process.

7. **Weight Drop:** Weight loss can occur as the body eliminates waste and toxins, particularly if there's lymphatic stagnation.

8. **Kidney Pain:** Kidney pain, often in the lower back or unexplained knee pain, can result from waste elimination. Adequate hydration is crucial.

9. **Headaches:** Frequent headaches often indicate elevated levels of toxicity in the bloodstream, commonly due to dehydration.

10. **Change in Taste & Smells:** Detox symptoms can affect your senses, causing changes in taste and smell.

These symptoms, while uncomfortable, are normal during

the body's cleansing process. They indicate that your body is expelling toxins and waste as it heals. Remember, proper hydration and sticking to your natural diet can help alleviate these symptoms over time.

As I mentioned, my headaches were frequent and severe for 20 solid years (age 15-35) and my poor grandmother suffered terribly having been diagnosed with skull cancer, she also suffered with head symptoms from dizziness, ringing in the ears and headaches.

I came across this quote written by Lauren Whiteman that I felt that I should include.

"Headaches are a big red flag and should be taken as an urgent warning sign. They are not a localized issue; they are communicating that the entire body is in distress due to its waste load. People with chronic headaches have a remarkably high risk of cancer and should heed the warning early and get their body back to suitable operating condition before it is too late." -- Lauren Whiteman

The time it takes to heal varies for each person due to individual factors. It is interesting because when you know you will eventually get better, does it really matter how long it takes? Healing is not like a specific moment; it is more gradual. One day, you realize you feel better, and that symptom is gone, even though you cannot pinpoint exactly when it happened. We might go through pain and discomfort, but later, it becomes a distant memory. You are fortunate because you have cut through the confusion about needing herbs or substances to heal. All you need is a commitment to a healthy life for your health to improve.

Chapter 16
Save the Planet: Heal Thyself

The journey to creating a better world starts with us. There is a lot of unnecessary suffering in the world, which could be easily alleviated with the right information and a willingness to make necessary changes. Nearly a decade ago, I hit rock bottom as my health issues and symptoms spiraled out of control. I was in constant pain, plagued by various ailments, and unable to fully engage in important moments in life. I regret missing out on significant moments with my children, spending most of my time battling headaches and only mustering the minimum effort for them before retreating to bed.

Regrets are unproductive, but if I were to harbor any, it would be about missing out on those precious moments. Fortunately, it was my pain that drove me to seek the information I've shared in this book. My situation was not unique; people everywhere are suffering, and illness is widespread. My unwavering determination to regain my well-being led me to the knowledge necessary to overcome debilitating pain and headaches. Deep down, I knew I shouldn't be in pain, and there had to be a better way. As I experienced my body's healing abilities, I began to understand the interconnectedness of everything. I realized that we could improve our surroundings on a micro level because everything is interconnected, and everything influences everything else. I witness this daily while working with nature.

I'm not the first to express these ideas, and I must admit that in the past, when I heard people talk about healing the world from within, it sounded somewhat "new age" to me. Our treatment of others often mirrors how we feel. When we feel good, the world appears promising, and we treat people well. When we're in pain or unwell, it's challenging to be our best selves, and it's unrealistic to expect peak performance when we're not feeling well. Food profoundly impacts our mood, affecting how we feel, function, and present ourselves.

For a significant part of my life, I never felt quite right. I was always ailing, preventing me from experiencing my true self or knowing what it's like to feel my best. However, at the time, I simply didn't know what I didn't know. Poor health hindered me from realizing my full potential, as it's challenging to focus on goals or have a vision when pain dominates your existence. I now understand that our interactions with others often reflect how we feel inside.

Some individuals excel at masking their suffering, but I'm not one of them. I can't fake a smile when I'm not feeling well. This is why strangers often told me to smile throughout my life. It reached a point where I wondered why I didn't smile as much as others thought I should. Looking back, I realize I didn't smile because I wasn't my true self yet. My pain frequently showed on my face and was noticeable.

To be honest, I feel like I'm just beginning this journey to a healthy life, and it's been nearly a decade. For ten years, I've exclusively consumed natural, health-promoting foods. This might seem like a long time, but when it comes to a complete lifestyle change and returning to the natural human diet, it's irrelevant. Once you embark on this path, the time it takes to heal and allow your body to correct itself becomes inconsequential, as you know that feeling better is inevitable; you just need patience. Nature accomplishes things in its own time, which cannot be rushed or predicted.

I often hear people say, "everyone is different," suggesting that some humans have unique dietary needs, like some being designed for meat consumption while others are not. However, we are one species, sharing a common design and functioning similarly on the inside. While we may reside in different parts of the world, natural fruits, greens, and vegetables are available almost everywhere, with only minor variations in variety. Regardless of where I go, I can find suitable foods to eat.

Unfortunately, our true history has been intentionally concealed from us. It would be more believable if we weren't saturated with lies and misinformation about our ancestors and our history. When we don't align our lives and diets with our body's requirements for optimal health, as most of us do today, we are at a disadvantage. Our bodies and minds cannot reach their full potential. We can argue about our species' exact dietary needs, but one thing is clear: most humans today are not in good health as a collective, and we can do better.

Heart disease is the leading cause of death, followed by cancer and medical errors. Despite these alarming statistics, we are somehow convinced that we are living longer and healthier lives. Through my work with numerous people trying to regain their health, I witness firsthand the immense suffering and the many individuals seeking non-conventional solutions for their health issues.

Pain can make us moody, and I have experienced this firsthand. When we don't feel our best, we can't be our best. Most of us strive to be positive and treat others with respect, but toxic behavior often stems from toxic individuals, contributing to the problems we face today.

It's clear that our collective toxic condition and behavior aren't solely due to food; factors like drugs, pharmaceuticals, vaccines, preservatives, geoengineering of our skies, food additives, and everyday toxic products all play a role. We are subtly under attack, and there's a silent war waged against us. However, the truth is, we allow much of it to happen. Most of what I mentioned is within our control, except for the chemicals being released into our environment. We can choose to avoid toxic foods and substances, but many lack knowledge about their harmful effects, and even those who do sometimes lack the willpower to avoid them.

Humans tend to choose the path of least resistance, but there's a price to pay. Consequently, most people are dealing with varying degrees of toxicity, often unaware because they don't know what they don't know. That's why the saying "just listen to your body" is only partly true. It should be "listen to your body when you're in good health." If we're still addicted to fast food, smoking, or an unnatural diet, we'll crave the same unhealthy foods we're accustomed to.

What we eat today influences our cravings tomorrow. A person who follows the natural human diet and has undergone periodic cleansing periods will naturally crave foods that benefit the body I can attest to this, having experienced both sides—the side wher I consumed a standard diet and my current unconventional diet.

In the past, my body was burdened with high levels of toxicity, leading to pain affecting my mood and behavior. My cravings were for foods that didn't serve my body. Today, I only crave foods that promote health and hydration.

During my time on the farm, I was merely surviving. The foods and substances I consumed suppressed my pain but allowed my health issues to progress. Most people find themselves caught in a vicious cycle of suppressing pain and symptoms through diets that demand substantial energy for digestion. When the body is continually overburdened with digestion, this cycle can persist for a lifetime, day in and day out. Taking short fasting breaks, for example, can make eliminations uncomfortable. Many people experience this uncomfortable sensation of digestive rest in the morning, leading to the popularity of large breakfasts that suppress these uncomfortable eliminations.

The sad truth is that when I think about almost everyone in my life and most people I know, I can hardly think of anyone who isn't suffering to some degree due to their life choices. Many people live in denial; they suffer, but because their symptoms are normalized and downplayed by society, they don't see them as significant issues. Pain and discomfort in the body, including headaches, irritability, mood swings, joint pain, brain fog, fatigue, digestive problems, constipation, memory issues, sleep disturbances, and other common symptoms, are not supposed to be part of the human experience. Everyone seems to be suffering, but ultimately, we inflict it upon ourselves.

Sometimes, I feel a deep empathy for people because something as seemingly innocent as our daily dietary choices can cause severe harm over generations. It seems unfair that we should suffer so much due to changes in our dietary choices across generations. Nature doesn't discriminate; if we don't provide our bodies with what they need to maintain health according to our original design, we inevitably suffer to varying degrees, influenced by unique factors in everyone's life. These facts sometimes feel surreal because not many people recognize them, and it's nearly impossible to do so unless we apply them and see how far removed we are from our natural dietary and lifestyle requirements. The notion of exclusively eating fruits, greens, nuts/seeds, and whole vegetables seems absurd and unimaginable to most people.

The few who choose to incorporate these healthy changes do so out of a desire to heal and live. They make these changes because they are suffering and, often in a poor state of health when they start, it takes time and patience to restore health. Unfortunately, many people lack the patience to wait; they are tired of pain and turn to pharmaceuticals or other remedies, further burdening their bodies.

I've heard people say they wouldn't want to live if they had to eat like me. It's a troubling sign when people are prepared to die for their food choices.

In a 2016 study, Johns Hopkins patient safety experts found that over 250,000 deaths occur annually in the USA due to medical errors. Medical errors rank as the third leading cause of death in the country, following heart disease and cancer. However, what's often overlooked is that for the medical system to be a leading cause of death, individuals seeking medical services are already dealing with serious health issues, often caused by their unhealthy diet and lifestyle choices. Hospitals, in my view, can be seen as "finishing houses"; they don't cause disease, but they may not necessarily help patients heal. Instead, they can either prolong suffering or worsen conditions with drugs and procedures. It may sound harsh, but it's essential to recognize that our choices, including what we eat and whether we seek medical care, are voluntary.

While the medical system can be invaluable during emergencies, such as accidents or broken bones, it may not always be the best solution for conditions that can be healed through simple diet and lifestyle changes. Taking medications for symptoms that could be resolved through these changes can lead to adverse outcomes.

Another aspect often overlooked is that patients who die from heart disease or cancer are frequently under medical care and advice. This means there's a chance that some patients may suffer from drug-related complications, even though the cause of death is attributed to their condition. People sometimes fail to realize that drugs can worsen their condition.

It's unfortunate that society tends to stigmatize those who deviate from the norm, such as individuals following unconventional diets like a high fruit raw diet or even a cooked food vegan diet. Such choices are often seen as eccentric or indicative of eating disorders or mental issues. This mindset is perpetuated by mainstream media, movies, magazines, and family traditions that prioritize cultural practices over health.

Many people struggle to understand that there may be alternative ways to live and that cherished traditions may not necessarily serve our health and well-being. Tradition should be adaptable and open to improvement, but it often resists change.

Personally, I've faced ridicule and rejection for my unconventional choices over the years. Whether I'm eating a watermelon in the park or filling my shopping cart with bananas and melons, people react with surprise and skepticism. People often make snap judgments based on brief observations, without considering that healing can involve moments when we don't look or feel our best. This can deter people from exploring healthier lifestyles.

What troubles me most is that my choices don't impose anything on anyone else. In fact, living in harmony with our natural needs requires less and doesn't intrude on others or the environment. Our natural diet is straightforward and doesn't require complex preparation. Still, because it isn't widely accepted, it's rejected by society as extreme.

While I'm confident in my choices and can withstand criticism, many people find it challenging to adopt a healthy lifestyle due to potential backlash. From my perspective, humanity's collective health is deteriorating, despite mainstream claims that we're living longer. Quality of life matters more than the number of years lived. Living a long life in constant pain without quality is a form of torture. I'd rather live fewer years with a high quality of life than extend my life while relying on others for care.

With each passing generation, our health seems to decline because we pass on weak and damaged genetics. Humanity may be on the brink of extinction unless more people wake up and actively work to reverse the damage. Our global issues won't improve when collective health continues to deteriorate.

The good news is that the body is resilient, even after decades of abuse, provided conditions haven't reached a degenerative stage. To see positive changes in the world and encourage people to improve in all aspects of life, we must start with ourselves. The state of the world reflects our internal condition, and our experiences are rooted in how we feel and our level of health. People don't harm others for no reason; they do it because they are damaged themselves. To initiate change, we must start with what we consume.

We are what we eat; our choices become us and shape our well-being. To build a better world, we must first focus on ourselves and embody the change we want to see. While it may sound cliché, it's the truth: we must become the change we desire for the world to change. I initially wanted to share what I learned about the true causes of disease and how to heal with everyone, but I was often met with resistance and rejection. Over time, I realized that people needed to see the positive changes in me before seeking my advice and knowledge.

A long time ago, I had a bumper sticker made for a family member. It had a somewhat vulgar message that said, "Save the planet, kill yourself!" Years later, as I was healing and transforming into a healthier version of myself, I started thinking about that bumper sticker. It struck me that it would make more sense (at least to me) if it said, "Save the Planet, Heal Thyself." This idea became the title not only for this chapter but possibly for this entire book, although I'm still considering it.

The core message is that we can't expect the world to change for the better if we're not willing to change ourselves. The world won't change on its own; it starts with personal transformation. My perspective on the world has shifted significantly since my health improved. The internet, which used to make me feel helpless about global issues, no longer has the same effect because I'm feeling stronger and healthier.

Our views and thoughts are closely connected to our inner health. Damage to organs like the liver and adrenal glands can affect our behavior, thoughts, moods, and outlook on the world, even if we're not fully aware of it. How we handle stress and our attitude toward life are also closely linked to our internal health. It's only when we step back and focus on our health that we can truly understand this connection.

Many people have no idea that something is wrong with their health because society has normalized common disease symptoms. People often accept how they feel as normal because it's all they've ever known, and gradual declines in health are seen as part of aging. They may never experience what true health feels like or realize what's possible for them.

I'll keep saying it: Food is mood. What we eat becomes an integral part of who we are on every level. I firmly believe I've discovered the root cause of human suffering: we're not creating the right conditions for health on a global scale. When humans suffer, everything around them suffers too, and we are supposed to be stewards of the land and all that surrounds us.

I hope to inspire you to explore a more natural diet if you haven't already. It's the first step to experiencing higher levels of health and contributing to a better world. Change begins and ends with you; it always has.

Before concluding this chapter, let me share the pillars of health that we need to focus on for optimal well-being. Anything valuable requires maintenance and care, and our bodies are no exception. While diet plays a significant role in shaping who we are, there are other pillars of health that work together with nutrition to build our overall well-being. Often, we tend to focus solely on one aspect, like nutrition or exercise, without considering health holistically. The truth is that all our essential needs play a crucial role in determining our overall health, and neglecting any of these needs can lead to imbalance and hinder our journey to optimal health. Our essential needs may seem simple and natural to meet in an ideal world. However, our reality is far from ideal, as we work long hours to sustain our lives, leading to unhealthy practices like prolonged sitting, limited exposure to natural light, lack of sunshine, reliance on less-than-ideal foods, unnecessary stress, and exposure to workplace chemicals. To navigate these obstacles, we must be proactive and knowledgeable about our health, identifying and overcoming challenges that society places in our path. Sometimes, this may involve letting go of negative influences, such as friends or family members who criticize or bring us down because of our unconventional choices. Achieving and maintaining health is no longer an easy path because few people are truly living well in today's world. Fast food restaurants are everywhere, so achieving health requires a strong desire for it and the ability to think creatively and make changes in our daily routines and lifestyle.

Today, our essential needs often get overshadowed in the flood of unnecessary and sometimes harmful health advice and information that dominates Western societies. The simplicity of meeting these needs may not seem impactful to the average person, which is why straightforward and beneficial dietary and lifestyle information often gets overlooked and dismissed. The Natural Human Diet is not a new concept; it has existed as long as humans have walked the Earth. Still, it hasn't gained much popularity among experts and the public. Several reasons contribute to this, including the addictive and satisfying nature of the foods most of us are used to, with harmful ingredients like salt, oils, artificial flavorings, and more.

Neglecting any of our essential requirements for health can lead to suffering and confusion, and I believe it's essential to share the other factors that must be met to achieve optimal health for our species. In today's world, it's convenient to disregard the laws of Nature with fast food on every corner, a pill for every ailment, and surgeries to buy us time. All this, combined with a lack of awareness of the true pillars of health, can prevent us from achieving the well-being we desire.

Below is an excerpt from The Life Science Course by TC Fry (lesson 3.1)

"When in a state of disease, most people do not realize they have brought it upon themselves. They are aided in placing blame outside themselves by a profession that takes the stance that they've had an unfortunate bit of bad luck, or they have been invaded by some microbial enemy. Though the needs of the ill differ from those of well people only in that their conditions must be made favorable to recuperation, both ill people and the medical professionals undertake a course of treatment that compounds sickness. Both the physician and the sufferer enter into an attempt to poison the ailing body back into health. The fact is that drugging only makes a body worse.

The causes of health are very simple. Our needs do not change substantially when we become ill. Even illness itself won't occur if the needs of our bodies and minds are properly met.

The nineteen factor elements for optimal well-being are listed as follows:

1. Pure air
2. Pure water
3. Cleanliness—both internal and external
4. Sleep
5. Temperature maintenance
6. Pure wholesome food to which we are biologically adapted
7. Exercise and activity
8. Sunshine upon our bodies
9. Rest and relaxation
10. Play and recreation
11. Emotional poise
12. Security of life and its means
13. Pleasant environment
14. Creative, useful work
15. Self-Mastery
16. Belonging
17. Motivation
18. Expression of the natural instincts
19. Indulgence of aesthetic senses." – TC Fry

It's important to take a moment to review each of the 19 points listed by TC Fry above and honestly assess where we stand in our own lives. We all face challenges, but it's crucial to keep striving for better health, not just for ourselves but also for our families and a world in need of healthy individuals more than ever. Save the planet, heal yourself!

 The good news is that people from all around the world are working to improve their health and lifestyle habits. The movement toward better health is growing, and with each passing year, more and more people are joining in to proactively care for their health and contribute to making our world a better place. I hope this book not only inspires you to gradually transition to our natural human diet but also provides valuable insights into the healing process and empowers you with the confidence and knowledge needed to become your own healer. Save the planet, heal yourself! Thank you for reading; I appreciate it.

Maria Manazza

The END

Printed in Great Britain
by Amazon

42309196R00116